Jane Brody's
ALLERGY
FIGHTER

Also by Jane Brody

Jane Brody's Cold and Flu Fighter

Jane Brody's Good Food Book

Jane Brody's Good Food Gourmet

Jane Brody's Nutrition Book

Jane Brody's *The New York Times* Guide to Personal Health

Jane Brody's Good Seafood Book (with Richard Flaste)

JANE E. BRODY

Jane Brody's
ALLERGY
FIGHTER

W. W. Norton & Company
New York London

For information about permission to reproduce selections from this book,
write to Permissions, W. W. Norton & Company, Inc., 500 Fifth Avenue,
New York, NY 10110.

The text of this book is composed in Bembo
with the display set in Berkeley Oldstyle Book
Composition manufacturing by The Haddon Craftsmen, Inc.
Book design by Chris Welch

Library of Congress Cataloging-in-Publication Data
Brody, Jane E.
[Allergy fighter]
Jane Brody's allergy fighter / by Jane E. Brody.
p.   cm.
Includes index.
ISBN 0-393-04059-3
1. Respiratory allergy—Popular works.   I. Title.
RC589.B76   1997
616.2'02—dc20   96-34499
CIP

ISBN 0-393-31635-1 pbk.

W. W. Norton & Company, Inc., 500 Fifth Avenue, New York, N.Y. 10110
http://www.wwnorton.com

W. W. Norton & Company Ltd., 10 Coptic Street, London WC1A 1PU

1   2   3   4   5   6   7   8   9   0

R0082761624

To Kris and Her Fellow Sufferers

Contents

ACKNOWLEDGMENTS

I consider myself very fortunate to have friends like Dr. Yalamanchi K. Rao. He is not only intelligent, perceptive, and the quintessential gentleman, but also a wonderful and patient tennis partner and an unusually fine physician. He is the kind of doctor who stays on top of his field—allergy—and always tries to educate his patients about their medical problems and the whys and wherefores of their treatment. Well-informed patients, he insists, adhere more closely to prescribed regimens and take better care of themselves.

Now, in the era of managed-care medicine, he is also deeply committed to teaching primary-care physicians the intricacies of allergy diagnosis and management. He knows that even if these physicians do most of the routine allergy care, there will always be patients who require the expertise of board-certified allergists.

His philosophy of well-informed patients and physicians fit handily with my request that he "examine" this manuscript for medical accuracy and thoroughness. This he did and much more. He provided piles of useful, up-to-the-minute background information. He answered my questions, complete with technical explanations, at all hours of the day and night. And he read, and reread, the manuscript, filling in gaps and correcting errors of commission and omission.

Dr. Rao—Kuchela—I could have done this without you, but not as quickly or as well. A "thank you" is hardly adequate.

—Jane E. Brody

Jane Brody's
ALLERGY
FIGHTER

Introduction

So You've Got "Hay Fever"

Would it make you feel any better to know that your condition is not caused by hay, nor is it a fever? Probably not! But the fact is, "hay fever" is one great big misnomer coined more than 150 years ago to describe the symptoms of ragweed allergy that are rampant in August and September, though it has gradually been extended to any and all pollen allergies. Pollen allergies attack through the nose and cause a host of symptoms—sneezing; runny nose; teary eyes; itchy eyes, nose, and throat, among others—that come and go with the seasons.

Hay fever is but one form of nasal allergy, a seasonal kind triggered by exposure to pollen. When you are allergic to something that you inhale continually or repeatedly regardless of the season, symptoms of nasal allergies can persist all year long. The symptoms of nasal allergies are caused by substances called allergens that float around in the air you breathe and play havoc with your immune system.

Literally hundreds of substances can cause nasal allergies. Most people with hay fever are sensitive to only one or a few, although some less fortunate souls seem to react to a dozen or more different allergens. The American College of Allergy, Asthma, and Immunology estimates that 75 percent of hay-fever sufferers are allergic to ragweed pollen, 40 percent are sensitive to grass pollen, and 9 percent react to tree pollen. However, 25 percent are allergic to both grass and ragweed pollen, and 3 percent are allergic to all three types of pollen.

As if that were not enough, many of these individuals are also sensitive to perennial allergens like dust mites, mold spores, and animal dander. They are likely to experience allergic reactions throughout the year, whenever they encounter these ubiquitous allergens. Just thinking about the problem of perennial allergies is enough to make an otherwise rational person want to stop breathing!

But no matter what is causing your symptoms, you'll be happy to know you need not go through life plagued by nasal allergies. Nor do you have to be "knocked out" by sleep-inducing antihistamines to quell your discomfort. Modern medicine has a host of solutions, ranging from avoidance tactics to non-sedating antihistamines to desensitizing injections, to help you control your allergies instead of them controlling you.

This book is designed to arm you and your family against the world of nasal allergens. Not only is there much you can do for yourself and others with allergies, you may also be able to help prevent allergies from arising in the next generation. Although nothing can guarantee that you'll never again have another siege of allergic sneezes, there is no question that you can—and that you deserve to—feel better than you do now. So, if your eyes are not yet too red and bleary, read on. . . .

1

AN ALLERGIC NOSE?
YOU ARE NOT ALONE

Your nose knows. It sneezes and sniffles, itches and twitches, gets stuffed and runs . . . and runs . . . and runs. Does it happen every spring? Late summer and fall? All winter long? All year? Then chances are you are among the more than 40 million Americans plagued by nasal allergies. Perhaps at first you think, almost hope, you've caught a cold. Colds, after all, are nearly always gone in a week. But allergies have a nasty way of hanging on for weeks or months (or sometimes all year), until the provoking substances no longer waft about in the air you breathe. And allergies, once they develop, can last a lifetime.

Alas, this is no cold. Colds don't tickle your mouth and throat or make your eyes itchy, red, and watery. Colds don't prompt you to think you should buy stock in a facial-tissue company. Colds don't get worse when you get a whiff of cigarette smoke or perfume or a strong-smelling household product or aerosol spray. And colds don't come on at the same time of year or under the same circumstances every year, year after year.

Does that jog or bike ride in May leave you feeling miserable instead of refreshed? Are you inclined to send your sinuses

to Arizona in August? Do you start sneezing or wheezing whenever you visit a friend who has a cat or a dog? Or when you
vacuum or dust? Or when you rent that summer cottage by the
lake? Or when you go down to the basement to find the camp-
ing equipment or holiday decorations? Or do your symptoms
kick in on Monday when you go to work, and subside over the
weekend?

If you answered yes to any of the above, you probably have
a nasal allergy, or, as physicians call it, allergic rhinitis. Your body
has a hyperactive immune system that overreacts to one or more
substances in the air as if they were mortal enemies. Among the
usual culprits are:

- Any of the dozens of types of pollen grains that fly about in
  search of a willing mate only to meet their demise in your
  nose.
- Mold spores spawned in dark, damp areas both indoors and
  out.
- Microscopic mites that dwell in house dust.
- The dander, saliva, urine, or feathers shed or spread by household pets or vermin, and the dusts, grains, or animals that people are exposed to on their jobs or through their hobbies.

In other words, nasal allergies can be seasonal, perennial, or
occupational. And as if these triggers were not trouble enough,
once a nasal allergic reaction is under way, any number of volatile
irritants—from smoke to fragrant soap—or even breathing cold
air can make you more miserable.

Plenty to Sneeze At

Half of the people with nasal allergies have symptoms for more
than four months of the year, and over 20 percent suffer for more
than nine months each year. Nearly a quarter of the children
who start off with seasonal allergies eventually develop year-

round allergic symptoms. Nasal allergies can render people of any age ultra-susceptible to respiratory infections like colds and flu, and prolonged allergy symptoms often set the stage for more serious complications, including asthma, sinus infections, ear infections, and nasal polyps.

Uncomplicated nasal allergies are not life-threatening the way a serious food or bee-sting allergy can be. However, they often exact a costly toll. Take seasonal allergies alone, which afflict nearly one person in ten and account for about half of all nasal allergies. A recent analysis estimated their annual cost at $2.7 billion in 1995 dollars. This includes direct costs: what sufferers spend on doctor visits, prescriptions, and over-the-counter medicines to curb their allergy symptoms; and indirect costs: time lost from work and reduced productivity resulting from allergic symptoms. Add on medical treatments necessitated by the complications of nasal allergies—chronic sinusitis, asthma, ear infections, and nasal polyps—and the costs of nasal allergies soar to an annual total of $10 billion.

But chances are, if you or a member of your family is a victim of nasal allergies, money is the last thing on your mind. Most prominent are the disruptive, discomforting, often embarrassing symptoms and the toll they exact on your quality of life. In addition to noses that run, itch, and get stuffed up, eyes that get red, itchy, and watery, and ears, mouth, and throat that itch, nasal allergies can cause sore throats, coughing, fatigue, stomachaches, headaches, and tenderness in the cheeks and forehead. Allergy symptoms can interfere with your participation in household and recreational activities, your ability to concentrate on your work or schooling, and your willingness to travel or visit other people's homes. Even in your own home, sleep is often impaired, headaches may make you tense and irritable, and you're likely to be chronically annoyed by the need to carry wads of tissues and repeatedly stop to blow your nose. As if all this were not disconcerting enough, the remedies people often choose to counter their allergic symptoms can make them sleepy and slow to react and dull their concentration and coordination.

That is the bad news about nasal allergies. The good news is that modern medicine has evolved effective weapons to counter them: to prevent symptoms from developing and to curb them when they do. Their proper use, however, depends greatly on an accurate diagnosis by the physician and acceptance by the sufferer of the measures necessary for any treatment to be fully protective. If you understand how allergies happen, you'll be more likely to follow your doctor's orders and reap the maximum relief.

2

HOW ALLERGIES HAPPEN

Allergies are a sign of an immune system run amok. Allergy symptoms result when an otherwise innocent substance—an *allergen,* which is almost always a protein—sets off a reaction that nature designed to protect the body from noxious invaders. In allergic rhinitis, the most common type of allergy, this reaction takes place in the mucous membranes that line nasal passages and surrounding tissues.

The main perpetrators of an allergic reaction are immune-system components called *mast cells.* Mast cells can be found throughout the body, but are most prominent in tissues that have contact with the outside world. Thus, the lining of the nose is replete with them, as are the skin and linings of the lungs, gastrointestinal tract, and reproductive tract. Every mast cell contains about 1,000 granules filled with *histamine* and other protective chemicals, which the cells can spew forth when danger threatens. Histamine, as any allergy sufferer who has taken an antihistamine probably realizes, is the chemical responsible for the bulk of allergy symptoms.

But before mast cells can release their supply of defensive

chemicals, something has to clue them in to the presence of a "threatening" allergen. That something is *an antibody called IgE, a specific type of protein produced by the immune system in response to a particular allergen.* Mast cells contain up to a million receptors for IgE antibodies. Receptors are like chemical locks into which only certain highly specific keys will fit. When someone prone to developing an allergy first encounters the allergen responsible, the immune system gears up by making IgE antibodies to that allergen. With each subsequent exposure, the body makes more and more of these specially programmed antibodies, and eventually there are enough to cause symptoms.

ANTIBODIES ON THE WARPATH

Symptoms result the next time this stockpile of programmed IgE antibodies encounters the allergen they were designed to recognize. The union of antibody and allergen triggers the underlying mast cells to release their granules and flood the area with histamines and other irritating chemicals, causing the runny nose and itchy eyes and throat that are classic symptoms of nasal allergies. It would be nice if once the mast cells released their arsenal, they would remain depleted. But no, within 6 to 24 hours the chemical-laden granules are fully reconstituted and poised to launch yet another attack in response to the allergen. And unlike most antibodies that last in the body for only a few weeks, IgE antibodies may hang around for years, and each time they encounter the allergen that triggered their production, they stimulate the mast cells to release symptom-inducing chemicals. And, of course, as old allergen-programmed IgE antibodies die off, the body will make new ones as long as you continue to be exposed to the allergen.

Let's say, for example, you are allergic to ragweed pollen, the leading cause of seasonal nasal allergies. You may recall from high school biology that pollen is the "sperm," or male half, of plant reproduction, and its task is to mate with a receptive female of the same species. On the surface of each pollen grain are enzymes that help it enter the female. When pollen gets inside the nose, the same enzymes are released. These enzymes, which are proteins, are the ultimate allergens that turn up production in the IgE factory. It usually takes about two to five seasons of exposure to an allergen like ragweed pollen before enough IgE is produced to cause allergy symptoms. Thus, people are not born with seasonal allergies. Rather, they gradually develop them, typically by adolescence or early adulthood but sometimes even in mid-life.

Now let's say you go off to live in Europe, where there is little if any ragweed. After many years, your body's pollen-sensitive IgE antibodies will die out. Then you come back to the United States, ragweed heaven. The first year or two, you'll probably feel fine during ragweed season. Then, slowly but almost certainly, your symptoms will return because, after all, your immune system has not changed; you had merely housed it in a less stimulating environment for a long time.

You may wonder why we have IgE antibodies in the first place if what they mostly do is cause misery. Their primary evolutionary function is to get rid of parasites that could cause serious illness. For as-yet-unknown reasons, in allergy-prone individuals IgE antibodies mistake innocent invaders like pollen enzymes and proteins in cat saliva for a declaration of war. And once the troops are unleashed, it is hard to rein them back in.

DELAYED REACTIONS, TOO

In fact, for about half the people with seasonal allergic rhinitis, the allergic reaction is not limited to their immediate exposure to an allergen. They don't just experience irritation from mast-cell chemicals. Rather, hours later white blood cells arrive on the scene and recruit still more irritating chemicals. This inflammatory reaction results in red, swollen, hot, and tender tissues that can prolong their misery for days, weeks, even a month following a single exposure to the allergen. With continued exposure to the allergen—for example, to the family cat—the combination of the immediate reaction and the delayed inflammatory response can perpetuate allergic symptoms indefinitely and create a fertile field for complicating infections or the development of asthma.

The delayed reaction also seems to prime a person's allergic sensitivity. As a result, the person may react more strongly to low levels of the allergen, or that person may react strongly to other allergens that previously had not been troublesome. Allergic priming also is believed to explain why nonspecific triggers like cold air or strong odors can cause allergy-type symptoms in many people.

Who's Allergic and Why?

How, you ask, did I become plagued by an overactive immune system that regards birch pollen or pussycats as mortal enemies? You may be able to start by thanking your parents. If either or both of your parents are allergic, you have a much greater chance of being so yourself. With two allergic parents, each child has about a 60 percent chance of also being allergic. With only one allergic parent, the chances drop to about 30 percent. But only about 10 percent of youngsters whose parents are allergy-free will themselves develop allergies.

Intense exposure very early in life to potential allergens like cats and irritants like cigarette smoke is also thought to increase a child's susceptibility to developing allergic rhinitis. Studies have also suggested that introducing an infant too soon to cow's milk or solid foods may foster an allergic tendency. The ideal food for babies for the first six months of life is breast milk, and if that is not possible, a special hypoallergenic infant formula. Even what mothers consume during pregnancy can affect their babies' chances of developing allergies to substances they inhale *(see page 74)*.

If one or both parents have allergic rhinitis, they would be wise to protect their babies from intense exposure to common allergens, especially dust, molds, and pets with hair or feathers.

It is important to keep in mind that allergies *develop*. You may be allergy-free all through high school, only to become unduly sensitive to airborne allergens while in college. For example, I experienced no symptoms while raising kittens as a young child. But at age twenty-three, while holding a Siamese kitten at a friend's house, I suddenly experienced a fit of sneezing, itchy eyes, and a nose that ran faster than I could catch it. Since then, I have had an unmistakable allergy to all cats, with a special sensitivity to Siamese.

Table 1 **Who Is at Risk?**

Allergic rhinitis rarely develops in a vacuum. Rather, certain factors increase a person's risk of developing a nasal allergy. You need not have been born allergic or predisposed to allergy. As the following list suggests, repeated exposure to allergens can eventually result in your becoming sensitive to them.

Environmental exposures to certain irritants also can increase your susceptibility to nasal allergy. This list should be treated as a cautionary note, not a cause for panic. Clearly, many people with even several of these risk factors do not develop allergies. Still, it would be wise for parents to do what they can to minimize the chance that their children will develop allergic rhinitis, especially if they themselves are allergic.

Genetic and Family Factors
Mother and/or father has allergies
One or both parents smoke
Poverty

Infancy Factors
Weighed less than 5½ pounds at birth
Born during peak pollen season
Exposed at an early age to cats or dogs
Exposed at an early age to natural-gas fumes
Born male
Not breast-fed
Given cow's milk or solid foods before 6 months

Exposures during Childhood and Beyond
Pollens
Animal dander
Molds
House dust mites
Latex
Cockroaches
Secondhand smoke

3

Do You Have
Allergic Rhinitis?

In medicine, determining the correct cause of a person's symptoms is often crucial to controlling them. That is particularly true for allergies. You may have good reason to suspect a pollen allergy if, for example, you get the same "cold" every May, or a cat allergy if your symptoms blossom whenever you visit your Aunt Tilly, who has two cats. And if your symptoms are not too severe and are adequately controlled by short-term treatment with an over-the-counter antihistamine, there may be no reason to see a doctor about them. If an antihistamine brings complete relief, that is, in effect, diagnostic of an allergy. And, unless you begin to develop complications or discomforting symptoms you cannot control, self-treatment can be medically sufficient.

However, for many people, allergic rhinitis is not that simple. Such people may be severely allergic to one thing or, more likely, sensitive to many allergens, not just one or two. And the antihistamines they can pick up in the drugstore may make them groggy but not significantly better. Furthermore, the triggers of their symptoms may be nearly impossible to avoid—unless they can survive without breathing or move to the moon.

Proper diagnosis and aggressive treatment are especially important in children who develop allergies early in life. In such youngsters, the allergies may progress to asthma or chronic ear infections that impair their ability to learn and to develop socially.

A proper diagnostic workup begins with questions about the patient's family history and exposures to potential allergens at home, at school, or at work, followed by a thorough physical examination of the nose, eyes, throat, ears, sinuses, and lungs. The doctor should ask when the symptoms occur, how severe they are, how long they last, and what circumstances—such as a change in the weather or exposure to cigarette smoke—make them worse.

Children and some adults with allergic rhinitis may have two telltale signs: a crease across the bridge of the nose caused by the infamous *allergic salute* (repeated rubbing of the nose in response to the running and itching) and dark circles under the eyes aptly called *allergic shiners.*

ALLERGY TESTS

If the patient's symptom history is not adequately revealing, skin tests may be needed to help pinpoint the allergic triggers. The results of these now-painless tests may reveal allergens that can be avoided, as well as those that might be countered by a series of desensitization injections. Such tests should be performed by a specialist in allergy—an allergist—who is equipped with emergency measures to counter a very rare but potentially dangerous severe allergic reaction.

Skin testing involves a series of tiny punctures or pricks on the skin after applying a drop of the various allergens likely to be encountered by the patient. Or tiny amounts of the allergens may be injected into the top layers of the skin, a technique called intradermal testing. At the same time, a skin test is done on the innocuous substance, such as salt water, that was used to dilute the test allergens so that the doctor can accurately interpret a person's reaction to each allergen. If the person is sensitive to an injected allergen, redness and slight swelling—called a wheal-and-flare response—will develop within 10 to 15 minutes at the site of the puncture or prick. The allergist can often tell how sensitive you are likely to be to a particular allergen from how strongly you react to it on a skin test. The redder and more inflamed the area becomes, the greater the likelihood that the allergen is also troublesome in real–world situations.

There are other ways to test for allergic sensitivity, though none is superior to skin tests and most are more expensive. The most popular alternative, called RAST (for RadioAllergoSorbent Test), is likely to be used when it is not practical or possible to do skin tests, such as when testing babies or people who take medications that would mask an allergic response. For RAST, the doctor takes a small sample of the patient's blood and places it in a machine that can measure the presence and amount of each type of IgE antibody the person harbors. If the test reveals a lot of IgE for ragweed pollen, for example, chances are the person is highly allergic to this pollen. Unlike skin tests, which give immediate results, you have to wait at least two days to get the results of RAST.

It is important for both patients and physicians to realize that a positive result on a skin test or RAST does not necessarily mean the particular allergen causes symptoms in real life. Just because you reacted to everything you were tested for to one degree or another does not mean you would react allergically to all those things if you inhaled them. It is also true that sometimes a skin test fails to detect an allergen to which you respond. Test reactions must be coordinated with a history of how the patient responds when exposed to the same allergens in daily life. Thus, you may react positively to a skin test for dog allergen, but when you are around dogs, allergic symptoms do not develop. Or an allergic response to dogs may occur only when you have already been "primed" through exposure to some other allergen you are sensitive to, such as ragweed pollen.

Table 2:   Classic Symptoms of Allergic Rhinitis

Nasal allergies can easily be confused with a cold or flu, since these ailments have certain symptoms in common. Many children and adults experience debilitating recurrent symptoms for years before someone suspects an allergy may be at the root of the problem. If some or all of the following symptoms occur often, it would be wise to ask a physician to explore the possibility that allergic rhinitis is their cause.

- Repeated sneezing
- Nasal itching and rubbing
- Nasal congestion
- Runny nose
- Dark circles under the eyes ("allergic shiner")
- Crease across bridge of nose (from "allergic salute")
- Frequent throat clearing
- Mouth breathing
- Diminished or lost sense of smell or taste
- Recurrent, unexplained nosebleeds
- Recurrent sinus infections
- Recurrent ear infections
- Cold-like symptoms that last more than 10 days
- Symptoms that recur at the same time each year

POSSIBLE COMPLICATIONS OF NASAL ALLERGIES

You may think that allergic rhinitis is little more than a nuisance. But this annoyance can sometimes develop into more serious health problems. That is why it is important to try to reduce your exposure and reaction to airborne allergens as much as possi-

Table 3:   **What Do You Have? Allergy, Cold, or Sinus Infection?**

Symptoms	Allergy	Cold	Sinusitis
Aching muscles	No	Often	No
Dizziness	No	Often	Sometimes
Dry cough	Sometimes	Often	Often
Fever	No	Often	Sometimes
Headache	Sometimes	Often	Sometimes
Hoarseness	Sometimes	Often	Sometimes
Itchy nose/eyes	Often	Seldom	Seldom
Discolored mucus	Sometimes	Often	Often
Unpleasant breath	No	Seldom	Often
Seasonal pattern	Often	Seldom	Seldom
Duration	As long as allergen is present	7 to 10 days	As long as infection is present

ble. These are some of the problems that may occur as a result of allergic irritation and inflammation.

Sinus Infections   When sinus cavities become inflamed, bacteria may grow in the fluid trapped in them, resulting in sinusitis, an infection that requires 10 or more days of antibiotic therapy. People who have repeated sinus infections should consider allergies as a possible reason for their susceptibility to this problem.

Nasal Polyps   Repeated swelling of nasal tissues in response to allergens can result in the formation of one or more small sacs, or polyps, inside the nose. Polyps can grow large enough to block air flow through that side of the nose. Once formed, they must be removed surgically.

What Should the Doctor Look For?

Symptoms and their timing do not always guarantee a correct diagnosis of allergic rhinitis. A thorough medical examination for possible allergy should include the following.

- Family and personal medical history, including information on environmental and occupational exposures.
- Description of symptoms, their duration and severity.
- Examination of the inside of the nose. Is the lining pale and swollen? Is there a polyp, foreign body, or deviated septum in the nose?
- Examination of the eyes. Are they puffy, red, and teary? Are there dark circles beneath them?
- Examination of the ears. Is there fluid in the middle ear or other signs of Eustachian-tube problems?
- Examination of the mouth and throat. Do they show signs of constant mouth breathing, such as a highly arched palate or elevated upper lip?
- Examination of the lungs. Is there wheezing or a persistent cough?

Conjunctivitis Also known as "red eye," conjunctivitis is an inflammation of the membrane that lines the inside of the eyelid and covers the white of the eye. Exposure to allergens can irritate the eyes and cause them to become red, itchy, puffy, and watery. Eyes may then be more susceptible to infection of the conjunctiva, which requires treatment with an antibiotic ointment.

Ear Problems Air flows in and out of the ear through the Eustachian tube, which connects the middle ear to the nasal passages. When this tube becomes blocked as a result of an allergic reaction, the air gets trapped inside and the ear feels plugged. Fluid may also build up in the middle ear and set the stage for an ear infection (serous otitis media) that requires treatment with

What Should the Doctor Ask You?

Any proper medical examination includes a personal history of factors possibly related to the patient's symptoms. Allergy experts say that a doctor should ask about the following matters when examining patients who complain of symptoms suggestive of allergic rhinitis.

1. Do either of your parents have allergies?
2. What symptoms do you have?
3. At what age did your symptoms begin?
4. When do the symptoms occur?
5. How long do the symptoms last?
6. How severe are the symptoms?
7. Do things like odors, weather changes, or stress cause the symptoms?
8. What kinds of furniture, carpeting, and bedding are in your home?
9. Do you have pets at home or at school? What kind?
10. Do the pets live indoors or out?
11. Do your symptoms get worse when you go to work and get better on weekends and vacations?
12. What medications—both prescription and over-the-counter—are you currently taking or using? Oral contraceptives? Thyroid hormones? Beta-blockers (see page 88)?
13. Do you regularly use a nasal spray or nose drops?
14. Do you smoke cigarettes, cigars, or a pipe?
15. Do you use intranasal cocaine, smoke marijuana, or use illicit inhalants?

antibiotics. Even without an infection, hearing may be impaired and the ability of the ear to equalize air pressure will be compromised, especially during descents in a plane, an elevator, or even in a motor vehicle going down a hill. The result can be a rupture in the ear. When serous otitis media affects an infant or

---

Quality-of-Life Checklist

In addition to assessing the severity of allergy symptoms, a physician examining a patient with allergic rhinitis should inquire about the effects of the ailment on the patient's quality of life. This can help the physician determine how aggressively to treat the patient's allergies and can provide a measure of the effectiveness of treatment. These questions were adapted from the "Rhinoconjunctivitis Quality-of-Life Questionnaire" developed by Elizabeth F. Juniper and G. H. Guyatt at McMaster University Medical Center in Hamilton, Ontario.

❑ **Sleep:** Do you have difficulty falling asleep? Do you wake up during the night? Do you awaken in the morning feeling unrested?

❑ **Emotions:** Do your symptoms cause you to become frustrated, irritable, impatient, restless, or embarrassed?

❑ **Nose:** How troubled are you by a stuffy or runny nose, sneezing, or postnasal drip?

❑ **Eyes:** How troubled are you by eyes that are itchy, watery, sore, or swollen?

❑ **Other symptoms:** Do you feel tired or worn out? Do you have frequent headaches? Do you have trouble concentrating? Do you feel poorly?

❑ **Practical problems:** How distressed are you by the need to rub or blow your nose or rub your eyes? Are you annoyed about always having to carry tissues with you?

❑ **Work:** Do your symptoms interfere with your ability to work at home, at school, or on the job?

❑ **Other activities:** Do your symptoms interfere with your ability to participate in athletic or recreational activities?

---

small child, impaired hearing can delay speech and intellectual and social development.

Asthma   This is the most serious of possible complications of nasal allergies. If the allergy causes irritation and swelling of the air passages in the lungs, breathing will become labored. A tendency to wheeze—for example, when exposed to nasal allergens or irritants or when exerting oneself—is a common symptom. Asthma can be a potentially dangerous and even fatal health problem that requires lifelong treatment. People with asthma should be under the care of a physician who specializes in treating this condition.

4

SNEEZIN' SEASONS:
SEASONAL ALLERGIC RHINITIS

"If it's May, it "must be . . ." could well be the signature phrase of someone with allergies to pollen shed by trees, shrubs, and grasses. Not every kind of pollen is a potential nasal allergen. To find its way into your nose, the pollen must fulfill certain criteria: it must be small and light enough to be carried by the wind, it must be produced in enormous quantities, and it must be found in places that people frequent. You may be surprised to learn that living in the city is not necessarily better for an allergic person than a rural area. In fact, air pollution in cities can prime a person for a more intense allergic response. And pollen can really get around, traveling as many as 20 miles to find a mate and encountering your nose en route.

Some 65 trees and shrubs, or one-tenth of the kinds that grow in North America, are capable of causing seasonal allergies. Among the common culprits are alder, ash, beech, birch, box elder, cedar, cottonwood, cypress, elm, eucalyptus, hickories, juniper, maples, mesquite, mulberry (the non-fruiting kind), oak, olive, osage orange, pecan, palm, poplar, sweet gum, sycamore, and willow. There is really no place to go to escape them all. The olive tree, for example, has become a terrible problem for allergy sufferers in Arizona, many of whom moved to that arid state to escape allergenic pollen in other parts of the country. Olive, cypress, juniper, and mulberry trees were planted widely in Arizona because they tolerate desert conditions well, but their pollen is highly allergenic. Olive-tree pollen is also a common nuisance to allergic people who live in southern California.

Also shedding pollen at about the same time many trees do are the grasses. Bermuda, blue, brome, canary, Johnson, orchard, redtop, rye, salt, Sudan, sugar beet, sweet vernal, timothy, and wild oats all produce highly allergenic pollen. And, again, there are only a few places—the desert and the frozen tundra—where you *might* escape them all. However, high concentrations of allergenic pollens from evergreens that live in subarctic regions manage to reach Greenland and Labrador. And even people in desert-like areas now have problems with grass-pollen allergies because so many communities have created 18-hole golf courses and yards planted with allergenic grass. Along with olive and mulberry trees, Bermuda grass is now a major allergy problem in southern Arizona.

Finally, there are the ubiquitous pollen-shedding weeds: greasewood, hemps, marsh elder, mugworts, nettle, pigweeds, plantain, rabbitbrush, ragweed, Russian thistle, sages, sagebrush, sheep sorrel, and smotherweed, among others.

INTERACTIONS WITH FOODS

As if the pollens themselves were not trouble enough, many foods contain proteins that are so similar to certain pollen allergens that they can intensify your reaction to pollen. You may think that ragweed is causing your late-summer misery. But before you place the entire blame on this highly allergenic plant, think about the cantaloupe, watermelon, or honeydew or the iced chamomile tea you found so refreshing at lunch, or the banana you sliced into your breakfast cereal. Any or all of these could be adding to your discomfort. Chrysanthemums and sunflowers also cross-react with ragweed, and in some people they will intensify the allergic response to ragweed. (See Table 4 on page 39 for clusters of food and pollen allergies.)

According to Dr. Leonard Bielory, director of the Allergy and Asthma Research Center at the New Jersey Medical School in Newark, cross-reactions between well-known allergens and certain foods are more common than most people realize. "Many people react to proteins that are found in all plants in the same family, and even if the plants are unrelated, there are some proteins they share that are basic to plant life," he explained. For example, an important transport protein called profilin, which was first identified as an allergen in birch trees, has since been found in latex (the rubber comes from a tree) and in a number of weed pollens.

Many allergists are concerned about the rising number of people who have become allergic to latex. Latex is the rubber used in most condoms and in surgical gloves now worn by health-care workers to protect against infectious viruses like hepatitis B and the human immunodeficiency virus (HIV) that causes AIDS. People with latex allergies have been reported to react to plant foods from a wide range of families: avocados, bananas, chestnuts, plums and peaches, potatoes and tomatoes, and kiwi fruit. Some also react to grass and ragweed pollens, melons, cucumbers, and squashes, whereas others have a cross-reacting allergy between latex and apricots, grapes, passion fruit, pineapple, figs, and papaya. Not only must such people avoid these individual foods, they must also take great care in consuming the mixed-fruit drinks that have become popular recently.

Table 4: **Allergen and Food Interactions**

Since many foods share allergenic proteins with pollens, people with pollen allergies may be wise to avoid certain foods during pollen season. Other allergenic plant substances, like latex, also interact with foods. And people with mold allergies may be sensitive to foods that are fermented or aged (and thus naturally contain molds). It may take some trial and error to determine which foods are a problem for you. These are some common "clusters" of possible allergen–food interactions.

If you are allergic to:	You may want to avoid these:
Ragweed	Bananas
	Cantaloupe
	Chamomile
	Honeydew melon
	Watermelon
Birch or Mugwort	Anise
	Apples
	Caraway
	Carrots
	Celery
	Coriander
	Cumin
	Hazelnuts
	Parsley
	Parsnip
	Peaches
	Peanuts
	Potatoes
Latex	Apricots
	Avocados
	Bananas
	Chestnuts
	Cucumbers

Figs
Grapes
Kiwi fruit
Papaya
Passion fruit
Peaches
Pineapple
Plums
Potatoes
Squashes
Tomatoes

Mold spores	Beer
	Buttermilk
	Cheese (especially aged)
	Cider
	Dried fruits
	Mushrooms
	Olives (cured)
	Pickled fish and meats
	Pickles
	Sauerkraut
	Vinegar and foods with vinegar

WHAT'S IN THE AIR NOW?

Just which allergenic pollens happen to be wafting by on local breezes depends on the season and geographical location. (Check Table 5 on page 41 for a national guide to seasonal allergies.) Because of climatic differences, a tree that is troublesome in April or May in the Northeast might be an allergenic culprit in February or March in the Southeast. In the Southwest, where peak allergy seasons cover eight months of

Table 5:   **Peak Allergy Seasons in Different Regions**

This table lists the times during the year when people allergic to seasonal allergens are likely to experience the worst symptoms. This doesn't mean, however, that someone who lives in the Northeast and has an allergy to grass pollen will experience no symptoms in March or July; in some years they might.

Region	March	April	May	June	July	August	September	October
Northeast	G G G G G G G G							
		T T T T T T T						
			W W W W W W W W W W W					
Southeast	G G G G G G G G							
		T T T T T						
			M M M M M M M M M M					
Midwest	G G G G G G G G							
		T T T T T						
			W W W W W W W W W W W					
Southwest			G G G G G G G G G G					
	T T T T T T T							
						M M M M M M M M		
			W W W W W W W W W W W W					
Rockies	G G G G G G G G G G							
		T T T T T T T T T T						
			W W W W W W W W W					
West		G G G G G G G G G G G G G G G						
	T T T T T T T T T							
			W W W W W W W					

Key: *G = grasses, T = trees, W = weeds, M = molds.*

the year, there is a brief (relatively speaking) hiatus in April, when every other part of the country is plagued by tree pollens. Remember, too, that it doesn't require a grove of trees or a field of weeds to cause allergy problems. A single pollen-shedding plant may liberate millions of pollen grains, any or all of which might be transported far and wide on the wings of the wind.

Many people wrongly blame showy flowering plants for their allergy symptoms. "Rose fever" is a common epithet for allergies that bloom in June, just when the roses do. But roses are pollinated by bees, as are most plants with ostentatious or fragrant flowers. Their pollen grains are too big and heavy to be distributed by the wind. Goldenrod, too, often gets blamed unfairly for the symptoms of ragweed allergy, which produces a far less obvious bloom at about the same time of year as goldenrod sends out its bright yellow stalks. Although goldenrod is a close relative of ragweed, its pollen is too heavy to be carried far from the plant. You would literally have to bump into it, or bring it into the house, to inhale the pollen.

Pollen Peaks and Valleys   Local weather conditions and daily patterns of air temperature, humidity, and wind speed all strongly affect how much pollen is likely to be in the air at a given time. Ideal conditions for transporting pollen are warm, dry days with briskly moving air. Thus, for most plants, peak pollen times are midday and afternoon, although some grasses favor early-morning or early-evening hours for their peak pollen release. In general, pollen counts at ground level peak between 8 A.M. and noon and again between 5 P.M. and 9 P.M. Between these times, when the sun is warmest, pollen tends to waft at higher elevations. So if you happen to live or work on the 20th floor and decide to open a window at 2 P.M., you may invite in a lot of pollen.

Short ragweed, the original cause of the misnomer "hay

fever," prefers to emit its pollen in the early daylight hours. However, the pollen grains usually do not reach urban areas in significant numbers until 2 to 4 hours later. This would mean that urban joggers with ragweed allergies might suffer least from an early-morning outing. Rainfall and fog around the time of sunrise suppress shedding of ragweed pollen, as do temperatures below 50°F (10°C). The large droplets that fall during a brief, violent thunderstorm are not effective air cleaners. But if a steady, gentle rain should happen to fall after the various trees, grasses, or weeds release their pollen, the air may be temporarily cleansed of these allergens. This would be another good time for the allergic to exercise outdoors (see also pages 45–51).

A Word about Pollen Counts

Many of those beset by allergy symptoms turn to the day's pollen count for a "see, I told you so" explanation for their suffering. But often these counts are close to useless, according to experts associated with the American Academy of Allergy, Asthma, and Immunology. At best, the counts may offer a clue as to why a person felt miserable *yesterday,* since all are based on pollen collected the day before.

The academy has promised that a new and more scientific system is on its way. While most published and broadcast pollen counts are now collected and analyzed in a haphazard manner, the academy is introducing a standardized system that could be used nationwide. The organization has established a national network of scientifically trained and certified pollen counters who report weekly to the home base in Milwaukee, where trends for the nation can be analyzed and correlated with weather patterns, climatic shifts, and changes in land use.

As of spring 1996, there were about 100 Academy-certified

pollen-counting stations throughout the country, all of them using standardized methods for collecting, analyzing, and reporting on pollen. The counts are also now being tabulated in a way that will make them more useful to allergists who are trying to help their patients cope better with seasonal allergies. When a patient is experiencing symptoms, the allergist can look at the current counts to see what pollens are prevalent that may account for the discomfort. The counts can also be used to monitor patients who are receiving allergy-desensitization shots to see how effective they are. And the counts can be reported to the local news media so that the public receives more accurate information.

Eventually, the academy hopes to use the standardized pollen counts to make predictions for the days ahead, instead of the Monday-morning quarterbacking that currently exists. Dr. Harriet Burge, an aerobiologist at the Harvard School of Public Health and manager of the national network, explained: "We hope to come up with predictive models based on what's happened historically. After we collect data for a few years, we should be able to use the historical record in a given area to predict the start of the various pollen seasons and even to predict which pollens will be around on which days, if it doesn't rain." As things stand now, an allergic person trying to plan the day's activities to minimize suffering would be better off listening to the weather forecast than to the pollen count.

Regardless of the specific counts, one fact is unmistakable: From early spring to late fall, most of North America is awash in an invisible rain of pollen. First it showers down from sunlit trees, then it flies up from drying grasses, and finally, toward the end of summer and through the fall until the first frost, it explodes from flowering weeds. Since we all have to breathe, we can't keep from inhaling airborne pollen. The culprits are floating everywhere, and we're just accidental intruders in the life cycle of plants.

"Bugged" by Allergies

In some parts of the country annual swarms of insects cause seasonal allergies in people sensitive to the body parts of these critters. As with plants shedding pollen, these insects have but one purpose—to find mates and produce the next generation to keep the species going. People just happen sometimes to get in the way. For example, around Buffalo, New York, large swarms of caddis flies are troublesome throughout the summer—June to late August—for those who happen to be allergic to them. And around Toledo, Ohio, airborne body parts of mayflies cause allergic reactions in June and July. The source of this misery? Lake Erie. This Great Lake harbors larval forms of these insects, and when they are fully developed they surface and fly to the shores, causing symptoms.

Of course, caddis flies and mayflies hatch in many other areas, where they are encountered not only by fisherpersons and those who navigate the waters where the larvae develop, such as the Mississippi River in Minnesota, but also by people who happen to live or play along the shores.

Exercising with Allergies

For someone with nasal allergies, the rapid or deep breathing induced by vigorous exercise is likely to invite in a whopping dose of airborne allergens that could negate the proverbial runner's high. But this need not be used as an excuse to stop exercising during pollen season. Nor should it force you to do your workout indoors during the nicest time of the year. Here are some protective measures that can help to keep you on the move all year long, regardless of what might be blowin' in the wind.

Just What's Bothering You?

Without sensitivity tests administered by a physician, you can't be certain about exactly what in the great outdoors is causing your allergic symptoms. Depending upon where you live, not only will the timing of airborne allergens differ, but so will the kind of pollen and the presence of molds. Here's what you might expect to encounter in different parts of the country. The listings reflect only the main, not all, offenders in each region.

The Far West
Grasses
Bermuda grass, Kentucky bluegrass, and rye grass in May through July in the eastern section, starting earlier and lasting longer along the coast. Bromegrass, rye grass, and Kentucky bluegrass in the San Francisco area from April through December and farther north along the coast from May to September.

Trees
Oak, poplar, and sycamore from January through May in the Northwest, February through May farther south, March and April in eastern Washington and Oregon. Olive trees in Fresno and southern California in February through May.

Weeds
Plantain and goosefoot; sagebrush around Reno and Los Angeles; dock and plantain from May through September in the Seattle and Portland regions; Russian thistle from July through October in southern California.

Molds
Alternaria in August and September.

The Southwest
Grasses
Bermuda grass, Johnson grass, and Kentucky bluegrass in May through September, longer around Phoenix and southern Texas, year-round around the Gulf of Mexico.

Trees

Cedar, ash, oak, and poplar from February through May; mulberry and olive from March through May.

Weeds

Tumbleweed, sagebrush, pigweed, burning bush, and saltbush from late June through September; saltbush from June through November in southern Texas; Russian thistle and ragweed in Oklahoma in August and September; amaranth in the Phoenix area from May through November.

Molds

Alternaria mid-August through October.

The Rockies

Grasses

Kentucky bluegrass, orchard grass, and redtop from May through August.

Trees

Box elder, birch, and poplar from mid-March through May.

Weeds

Russian thistle, sagebrush, and false ragweed from August through mid-October, though Russian thistle sometimes starts in May.

Molds

Alternaria in August and September.

The Plains States

Grasses

Kentucky bluegrass from May to perhaps July.

Trees

Oak, box elder, alder, ash, birch, and sycamore from March through May.

Weeds

Ragweed in August and September, with an earlier start in North Dakota; Russian thistle and amaranth in Kansas from July through September; sagebrush in the Dakotas from mid-August through September.

Molds

Alternaria spring through fall.

The Midwest
Grasses
Kentucky bluegrass, timothy, orchard grass, and redtop from May to mid-July.
Trees
Oak, poplar, walnut, box elder, and ash from March through May.
Weeds
Ragweed in August and September.
Molds
Alternaria in August and September.

New England
Grasses
Kentucky bluegrass and timothy from May through July.
Trees
Birch, oak, sycamore, willow, hickory, and maple from mid-March through May.
Weeds
Ragweed and amaranth from mid-August to late September, except no ragweed in northern Maine.
Molds
Alternaria in August and September.

Mid-Atlantic States
Grasses
Kentucky bluegrass, redtop, timothy, and salt grass from May through July.
Trees
Oak, birch, hickory, walnut, maple, and sycamore, among others, from March through May, starting earlier and ending sooner in the southern states.
Weeds
Ragweed, goosefoot, pigweed, and plantain in August and September.
Molds
Alternaria in August and September.

The South

Grasses

Bermuda grass, Kentucky bluegrass, Johnson grass, orchard grass, and wild rye from May through September, through August in the Carolinas, from April through November in Louisiana, year-round in subtropical Florida.

Trees

Oak, sweet gum, pecan, box elder, ash, and cottonwood starting in mid-January in Georgia and in March in Kentucky until the end of May.

Weeds

Ragweed, marsh elder, pigweed, and goosefoot from August through September in Kentucky, Georgia, North Carolina, and Florida (sometimes starting in June in southern Florida), and extending until October or November in South Carolina, Tennessee, Louisiana, and northern Florida. Sagebrush in Tennessee in September.

Molds

Year-round except where temperatures drop below freezing.

- Try to schedule your outdoor exercise time when pollen counts are likely to be lowest. This means just before or after daybreak, before the sun dries the pollen-bearing anthers and the morning breeze picks up and distributes those pesky pollen grains. Another good time might be in mid-afternoon when pollen tends to ride high in the air, or after sundown when the breeze dies down and pollen grains descend to the ground.
- Pay attention to the weather. The best days for outdoor exercise are likely to be those that are cloudy or chilly, humid, and windless or very windy. Pollen counts are lowest during or after a steady rain.
- Choose your location wisely. Running through the woods when the trees are pollinating or through the fields when

grasses and weeds are shedding their reproductive wares is simply inviting trouble. Stick to paths that are well-worn and away from troublesome vegetation. But also try to avoid areas near heavy vehicular traffic; the air pollution will increase your sensitivity to any allergens you happen to inhale.

- Consider wearing a pollen-filtering mask over your nose and mouth and goggles or wraparound glasses to keep as much pollen away from your mucous membranes as possible.
- To reduce the amount of time you spend inhaling pollen and pollutants, do your warm-up indoors. An indoor warm-up is especially helpful in cold weather for people who tend to develop asthmatic symptoms when they exercise.
- About half an hour before your workout, take an antihistamine or decongestant, or a combination of the two. Helpful medications are available over-the-counter and with a physician's prescription (see pages 80–108). The new antihistamines that do not cause drowsiness currently require a prescription.
- Prior to your workout, use the prescription nasal spray cromolyn sodium, which helps to prevent an inflammatory response to nasal allergens (see page 89). There are also prescription and over-the-counter eye drops that can help protect against red, itchy, watery eyes (see page 92).
- If during peak pollen season your symptoms become severe, cortisone sprays, available by prescription, can bring relief (see page 90).
- If you are severely allergic and find that your symptoms are keeping you from enjoying your favorite activities, consult your physician about getting desensitizing injections (allergy shots; see pages 109–12).
- If all else fails, you might consider moving your workout indoors during the worst of the pollen season. Health clubs and Y's throughout the country offer interesting options: step classes, water aerobics, strength training, swimming, station-

ary cycling, treadmills, cross-country ski machines, running tracks, and so on. Many have one-month and three-month memberships, which should get you through the peak pollen season.

GARDENING WITHOUT TEARS

The fact that you or a member of your household suffers from pollen or other inhalant allergies need not keep you from putting in and maintaining lovely landscaping around your home. Though it may seem as if you're allergic to the world of blooms, there are actually far more trees, shrubs, and flowers that are unlikely to provoke allergies than are likely to cause you discomfort. In fact, it may delight you to know that plants with the showiest blooms, including roses ("rose fever" is a misnomer), are nearly all pollinated by insects, not wind, and so are not a source of nasal allergens.

While outdoors, you are likely to breathe in hundreds of pollen grains every second. But you can minimize your exposure by planting trees, shrubs, and flowers with little or no potential for triggering nasal allergies (see Table 6 on page 53) and by keeping the grounds around your home well-maintained and free of flowering weeds. Highly allergenic weeds include ragweed, mugwort, cockleweed, dock, English plantain, lamb's-quarter, pigweed, sagebrush, amaranth, and Russian thistle.

You can reduce pollinating weeds, dust, and mold spores by using black plastic to mulch your vegetable garden instead of straw. In addition to greatly reducing weeding chores, the plastic helps to warm the soil and reduce evaporation. Watering the soil regularly with a sprinkler can keep down dust and reduce the amount of mold spores that become airborne.

To prevent grasses from flowering and shedding their pollen, keep the lawn trimmed as short as possible (no longer than 2 inches). If possible, hire someone else to cut the grass and weeds and do the yardwork. But if you must—or you prefer to—do it yourself, wear a protective mask, gloves, and goggles or wrap-around glasses. Keep your hands off your face while you're working. As soon as you're done working outdoors, remove your clothing and put it in the wash, then shower and wash your hair.

If possible, do your gardening on cool, cloudy, humid, windless days or just after (or even during) a steady rain, when the pollen count is likely to be lowest. Also consider taking an antihistamine before doing any extended gardening that is likely to expose you to allergens to which you react.

Think twice before bringing fresh blooms into your house, even if they seem to be trouble-free while in the garden. Safest are the flowers that bees hover around, such as roses and bee balm; these have pollen too heavy to become airborne. However, you might want to choose flowers that emit no perfume, since some people are sensitive to flower scents, especially when their allergies have already been triggered by true allergens.

In general, if someone with nasal allergies is present, it is unwise to bring flowering weeds into the confines of a home. Though they may not seem troublesome when diluted by the air of the great outdoors, more intense indoor exposure could trigger symptoms.

Table 6:   **What to Plant**

While you can't keep your neighbors from growing trees, plants, and weeds that trigger your allergies, you can at least reduce your exposure by landscaping sensibly on your own property. If you or any member of your household has nasal allergies, you would be wise to consider the following.

Avoid plantings with a high allergenic potential, such as these trees and shrubs . . .

Ash	Olive
Birch	Pecan
Cottonwood	Poplar
Cypress	Privet
Elm	Red cedar
Hickory	Sweet gum
Juniper	Sycamore (London plane)
Maple	Walnut
Mulberry (non-fruiting)	Willow
Oak	

. . . and these plants and grasses:

Amaranth	Redtop
Artemisia	Sorrel
Bermuda grass	Sweet vernal
Bluegrass	Timothy
Orchard	

Instead put in plantings with low allergenic potential, such as these trees and shrubs . . .

Apple	Maidenhair (ginkgo)
Azalea	Oleander
Boxwood	Palm
Catalpa	Pear
Cherry	Pine
Dogwood	Plum

Fir
Fruited mulberry
Hawthorne
Hibiscus
Hope chestnut
Magnolia

Pyracantha
Redbud
Silk tree
Tulip tree
Yew
Yucca

. . . and these flowering plants and grasses:

Allium
Azalea
Begonia
Bougainvillea
Cacti
Columbine
Coneflower
Crocus
Daffodil
Dahlia
Dichondra
Geranium
Gladiola
Hollyhock
Hyacinth
Impatiens
Iris
Irish moss

Larkspur
Lavender
Lilies
Marigold
Orchids
Pansy
Peony
Periwinkle
Petunia
Poppy
Ranunculus
Rose
Salvia
Tulip
Verbena
Vinca
Violet
Zinnia

5

WHEN THE MISERY PERSISTS: PERENNIAL ALLERGIC RHINITIS

So it's the dead of winter and you think the allergy season is, or should be, over. How, then, do you account for that "cold" that seems to be hanging around for months—the runny or stuffy nose, sneezing, postnasal drip, irritating cough, and itchy throat that don't go away and stay away even though all pollinating plants are now dormant? There's a good chance you are a victim of a winter allergy, or, as it is called medically, perennial allergic rhinitis.

Those with only pollen allergies are, in a sense, lucky. Their suffering is limited to the mating season for the plants to which they're sensitive. Others less fortunate experience allergy symptoms virtually all year to a greater or lesser degree. Their immune systems regard substances commonly encountered at home or at work—such as dust mites, mold spores, and animal dander—as major threats, and launch repeated attacks against these nearly ubiquitous contaminants of the air we breathe.

Those with perennial allergic rhinitis who are also sensitive to pollens simply get worse during pollen season. In fact, perennial allergies can exaggerate a person's reactions to seasonal pollens, delivering a double-whammy to those with spring and fall allergies. And people with perennial allergies seem especially prone to developing chronic ailments like sinusitis, fluid in the middle ear, bronchial hypersensitivity, or even asthma triggered by persistent upper respiratory congestion or postnasal drip.

MITES, MOLDS, AND OTHER PERENNIAL ALLERGENS

The three most common causes of year-round allergies are the excrement of microscopic mites that live in house dust, spores released by molds that grow in dark, damp areas indoors as well as out, and the saliva of household pets, which contaminates their hair, skin, or feathers when the animals clean themselves. There are other less savory sources of perennial allergens, like the body parts of cockroaches and the urine of rats and mice that prefer your cozy dwelling to the cold, cruel outdoors. Of course, rats and mice are not the only "household" rodents with allergenic urine. How about those popular animals—hamsters, gerbils, guinea pigs, and rabbits—chosen as pets for many young children and classrooms? (After all, they don't have to be walked!)

Mites and molds thrive when their surroundings are warm and moist. They prefer temperatures above 70°F and a relative humidity above 50 percent. That would make the summer months their most prolific time of year. You might expect them to die out during the winter heating season, when indoor temperatures are commonly cool and the indoor air is often drier than the Sahara Desert. But, alas, many mites and molds do quite well indoors all year long, and sometimes the very measures people take to relieve winter dryness make matters worse. The problem of indoor allergens has been aggravated by attempts in recent decades to create "tight" dwellings to conserve fuel and reduce utility costs. The less the air circulates, the more contaminated it can become, and with windows and doors tightly closed all winter, a home can become a hotbed of perennial allergens.

Dust Mites   No matter how meticulous a housekeeper you may be, your living quarters will still play host to millions of dust mites. Each female mite can lay 25 to 50 eggs and produce a new generation of mites every three weeks. These microscopic animals live on tiny bits of organic matter—mostly scales shed by human skin—that are present in dust, and they produce waste particles that are the ultimate allergens. Each mite produces about 20 such particles every day; even long after the mite that produced them has died, the waste particles can continue to provoke allergic reactions.

Dust, and therefore dust mites and their excrement, is everywhere: in rugs and carpets, in mattresses and pillows, in files and piles of papers, on bookshelves and under furniture, on window blinds, curtains, and drapes, on stuffed animals, dried flowers, and knickknacks. Every step you take on a carpet or rug sends a cloud of dust—and dust-mite allergen—wafting into the air you breathe. Every time you lie down in bed or alight on upholstered furniture, another mini dust cloud rises to greet you. And unless you take special precautions to prevent it, every time you vacuum or dust the furniture, dust-mite allergen is spewed into the air as if you'd sprayed it from an aerosol can. (See pages 68–71 for steps you can take to reduce exposure to dust mites.)

Mold Spores   Molds are microscopic fungi (perhaps you call them mildew) that live on plant and animal matter. They thrive in bathrooms, basements, garages, and crawl spaces, under sinks, in refrigerator drip pans and garbage pails, on wallpaper, behind washing machines and freezers, in humidifiers and air conditioners, and on damp walls, floors, and window ledges. A carpet laid over an unprotected concrete floor is a perfect breeding ground for mold because moisture can seep up through the floor. Piles of leaves, the bark on fireplace logs, compost heaps, garden soil, and debris-filled rain gutters are favored outdoor sites for molds to colonize. Drainage problems around or under the house—or even on the roof—could foster mold growth indoors. Other favored mold environments include greenhouses, antique shops, sleeping bags, summer cottages, hotel rooms, and automobile air conditioners.

Some workers are heavily exposed to molds in the course of their work, among them gardeners, farmers, carpenters, plumbers, brewers, florists, upholsterers, paper hangers, book handlers, and furriers.

Molds reproduce by emitting spores, which are released into the air when the spores mature and whenever the colony of molds is the least bit disturbed. Just the breeze created by walking past a moldy site could aerate spores that are ready to be released. Reorganizing things in the basement or cleaning out the garage could result in a shower of mold spores. And preparing the garden for spring planting, or turning over the compost heap, can expose you to uncountable millions of these reproductive bodies. Even during the worst allergy season, airborne mold spores are likely to be far more numerous than pollen grains. (See pages 65–68 for tips on reducing your exposure to mold spores.)

Pets and Other Animals   An allergy to a pet is perhaps the hardest to take. Pets are often among the most loved members of a family, and parting with a pet because someone in the family is allergic to it is likely to make everyone miserable. Contrary to popular belief, the actual allergy is not to the animal's hair, feathers, or shed skin but to proteins in the saliva. Animals that clean or preen by licking themselves cover their coats with these proteins. This is one reason why many more people are allergic to cats than dogs. Actually, a person may be equally allergic to both, but only cats provoke symptoms because cats spend more time cleaning themselves and in the process coat nearly every hair and millimeter of skin with their saliva. These allergenic proteins are tiny—smaller even than the waste particles of dust mites—and easily become airborne throughout homes that house cats. Cat allergen can contaminate every bit of upholstered furniture in the house, the carpets, the mattress and bedding, even the walls.

Keeping away from the cat or keeping the cat outside the bedroom of the allergic person is rarely adequate protection if the cat lives in the house. Cat allergen can easily spread everywhere through the duct system in homes heated by hot air. Cat allergen is also sticky and readily clings to the clothing and skin of whoever handles the animal; that person can then transport the allergen everywhere. In fact, many people with cat allergies will develop allergic symptoms just from sitting near or working with someone who owns a cat. (See pages 71–74 for advice on "safe" pets and pet-keeping practices for the allergic.)

As previously mentioned, other animals—uninvited household guests like roaches and rodents, and rodents that are kept as pets—can also cause allergic rhinitis. If the rodent-control products you can buy in the supermarket or hardware store are not able to rid your home of allergenic vermin, call an exterminator. If the troublesome rodent is a pet, consider replacing it. If that is not acceptable, keep the animal in its cage at all times, keep the allergic person away from it, and do not allow that person to clean the cage.

Occupational Rhinitis

Many of the substances that make workers sick are not, strictly speaking, allergens because they cannot stimulate the production of IgE antibodies. Rather, they are irritants or fumes, such as volatile chemicals, smoke, formaldehyde, and mineral dust. And many of the workers who are sickened on the job do not handle toxic or irritating substances; they are office workers who breathe foul air, including dust-mite allergen, that permeates the tight, improperly ventilated buildings they inhabit for eight or more hours a day, five days a week. Still, the symptoms they suffer are often indistinguishable from perennial allergic rhinitis and, as far as affected workers are concerned, they are "allergic" to something at work.

A worker sensitive to nonallergenic irritants has limited choices: get the boss to clean up the work environment by installing effective filters and other antipollution devices; wear protective clothing (including a filtering face mask), or find another job.

The most common on-the-job nasal allergens are mold spores, dust mites, roach parts, laboratory animals, and pollen grains that can permeate a work environment. There are a few occupational chemicals—such as quarternary ammonia compounds—that are enough like proteins to allow them to serve as allergens and trigger the production of IgE antibodies. In addition, some reactive chemicals encountered by workers are capable of transforming themselves into allergens by hooking up to proteins in the body. (See Table 7 on page 61 for a list of common occupational causes of allergic rhinitis.)

Table 7: **Allergic Rhinitis on the Job**

Workers can be exposed to literally hundreds of substances that cause respiratory symptoms. Most are not allergens. For example, a runny or stuffy nose can result from exposure to the strong odors of tobacco smoke, fragrances, cleaning agents, and exhaust fumes, or from irritants like formaldehyde, paint fumes, ozone, and other air pollutants. Sometimes corrosive substances like ammonia, chloride, certain pesticides, and acrylamide used in plastics manufacturing are the culprits. Still, there are plenty of other substances that provoke a true allergic reaction, complete with the development of IgE antibodies to the offending substance. These are potential allergens that millions of workers are exposed to on their jobs. Of course, if the allergic worker is also exposed to strong odors, irritants, or corrosive substances, the reaction to the allergen can be much worse.

Allergen	Occupational Environment
Animal proteins	Animal laboratories, pet stores, bee farms
Wheat	Food-processing plants
Green tea	Processing/packaging plants
Pyrethrum	Fumigant, insecticide, and gardening industries
Cotton fibers	Cotton mills
Reactive dyes	Textile industry, beauty salons
Toluene diisocyanate	Autobody spray painting
Trypsin	Drug, chemical, and plastics industries
Papain	Meat-processing plants, breweries
Latex	Health-care industry
Platinum salts	Jewelry and refining industries
Colophony	Metal and electronics industries
Acid anhydrides	Adhesive and plastics industries
Plicatic acid	Cedar sawmills

6

AVOIDING THE CAUSES
OF ALLERGIC RHINITIS

An ounce of prevention, it is said, is worth a pound of cure. This is as true for nasal allergies as it is for infectious illnesses that can be prevented by a vaccine. While you may not be able to eradicate your allergies or the substances that trigger them, you can often do a great deal to minimize your exposure and symptoms. Avoidance tactics may enable you to get along well without allergy-squelching medications or repeated visits to a physician for desensitization shots. (See pages 126–27 for purchasing information about the products discussed in this chapter.)

POLLEN

Allergy symptoms that occur only in the spring or late summer and fall are most likely the result of inhaled pollen. The timing and specific causes will depend primarily upon where you live (see Table 5 on page 41) and, to a lesser extent, on the local weather. The troublesome pollen grains will be in the air no matter what, so your goal is to inhale as few of them as possible.

When Traveling   Keep the windows closed in the car and use the air conditioner (on "recirculate," if that setting is available). And be sure to have the air conditioner serviced regularly to remove the accumulated molds and dust. Take the scenic route through back roads instead of congested highways to reduce the pollutants you inhale, which can aggravate nasal allergies.

If possible, during peak pollen season plan trips to someplace relatively free of the pollens that plague you—for example, someplace hot and dry like the Southwest desert or at the shore where sea breezes tend to keep the air pollen-free. Or you might head for the hills; mountain ranges that exceed 5,000 feet tend to have fewer airborne allergens. For those with ragweed allergies, Europe would be an excellent vacation spot.

However, if you're thinking of escaping a northern winter by heading south, keep in mind that allergy season is year-round in subtropical and tropical areas. One New Yorker I know who spends part of each winter in Florida (to please his wife) is miserable for the entire time because of pollen allergies.

Outdoors at Home   If you cannot get away from it all by taking a vacation during pollen season, try to reschedule your outdoor activities to minimize the amount of pollen you inhale. The best defense against pollen, as with most aggressors, is to stay out of the line of fire as much as possible. Try to stay indoors in an air-conditioned area during the hours of the day when airborne pollen is at its peak. Pollen is least likely to be in the range of your breathing passages during the night, at daybreak when plants are still covered with dew, during and after a steady rain, and on cloudy, humid, windless days. High winds, too, reduce the pollen in the air.

Even on those warm, dry, and breezy high-pollen days, some

times are better than others. Try to do your outdoor exercise during the early-morning hours—say, between 6 A.M. and 8 A.M. in spring and even earlier in summer—before the sun is high and hot enough to dry pollen-bearing anthers and prompt them to shed their wares. Another relatively low pollen period is usually mid-afternoon on a hot, sunny day when hot air currents carry pollen high into the air and out of reach of your breathing zone.

Consider wearing goggles, or at least wraparound glasses or sunglasses, when going outdoors in pollen season. Though not exactly glamorous, a pollen-filtering nasal mask can help protect those who are highly sensitive to pollen. The masks, which resemble surgical masks, are available in drugstores. At the least, wear a pollen-filtering mask when mowing the lawn or doing any kind of yardwork. Mowing and raking stir up enormous quantities of pollen, not just grass pollen but also tree pollen that has fallen to the ground.

Minimize the amount of pollen you bring indoors. After spending time outdoors, if you were wearing a jacket, remove it before entering the house and shake it out. Then shower, wash your hair, and change clothes to avoid continued exposure to the pollen that clings to you and your clothing. If possible, hang your clothes someplace other than in your bedroom closet.

If you have pollen allergies, use a clothes dryer. As fresh as the laundry may smell after drying on an outdoor line, it will also be laden with pollen.

Breathe Clean Indoor Air   Keep your home environment relatively pollen-free by shutting doors and windows. Again, use an air conditioner to cool the air and filter out some of the airborne pollen. If you get a special filter for your air conditioner, it will remove nearly all the allergenic particles. The filter is called HEPA, for *h*igh-*e*fficiency *p*articulate *a*ccumulator. If you have no air conditioner, consider using a freestanding electric HEPA air filter in your bedroom and the rooms where you spend most of your waking hours. An effective filter can be purchased for $100 or less.

Avoid Irritants   Air pollutants and strong odors can enhance the symptoms of pollen allergies. At least during the time your symptoms are at their worst, avoid wearing perfumes, colognes, and scented lotions. Nearly every cosmetic product is now available in a scent-free form: deodorants, skin creams, lipsticks, hair sprays, soaps, etc. There are also unscented laundry detergents. If it becomes necessary to use an irritating substance, try to find someone else to apply it for you and leave the area until the odor dissipates. If needed, HEPA air filters are also effective in removing odoriferous particles from the air. Potpourris, which some people use to "freshen" the air in bathrooms and bedrooms, are my particular nemesis. Perhaps they are yours, too. If so, get rid of them—fast!

MOLDS

Mold allergies can be bothersome almost any time of the year, both indoors and out. You can reduce your discomfort by controlling mold growth in your living quarters and spending as little time as possible in mold-ridden areas or doing activities that stir up mold spores.

Avoid Moldy Areas   Basements, garages, crawl spaces, barns, compost heaps, woodpiles, and blankets of fallen leaves tend to be breeding grounds for molds. If you must be exposed, wear a face mask. Other environments that are commonly mold-ridden include antique shops, pool areas, and summer cottages that are shut down all winter. Even automobile air conditioners may harbor molds, creating a dilemma for those allergic to both pollen and molds.

Keep the Humidity Down   The humidity in your home should be kept below 40 percent to discourage mold growth. Monitor it with a gauge. Use air conditioners and dehumidifiers when the humidity is high—usually during the summer months. Consider installing a dehumidifier in damp, enclosed areas like the basement. Avoid overhumidifying the air during the winter; 35 percent is high enough. If the outer walls and windows of your home are getting wet, the humidity is too high; mold will grow on the damp surfaces.

Use an exhaust fan over the stove and in the bathroom to remove excess humidity generated by cooking and showering. Don't put damp clothes or shoes away in closets or drawers. Let them air out and dry completely first. Vent the clothes dryer to the outdoors, and don't leave wet clothes lying around for hours in the washing machine. If necessary, set a timer to help you remember to put the clothes in the dryer as soon as the washer stops. If you must hang wet clothes in the house, consider buying a portable dehumidifier for the area.

Control Trouble Spots   Refrigerators commonly breed molds—on the gasket around the door, in the water pan under a self-defrosting unit, and on foods that are forgotten and left to spoil. Clean the refrigerator and empty the water pan regularly and discard spoiling food promptly.

Regularly wash shower curtains and bathroom tiles, grouting, and fixtures with mold-killing and mold-preventing solutions, such as Lysol or a bleach solution. Use only machine-washable bath mats, not carpeting, in the bathroom. After leaving the shower, stretch out the curtain to deter mildew.

Don't overload your house with live plants. Wear a mask if you must dig around in the soil or transplant houseplants, which stirs up molds that live on the soil surface. Immediately empty the water that seeps into the saucers under plants when they are watered (it's no good for the plants either!). Dried flowers also often contain molds. If you decorate for Christmas, avoid bringing a live tree or wreaths into the house. If you have a fireplace, store firewood outdoors.

If the house is damp and always shaded by vegetation, prune trees and bushes often and perhaps have some of the trees removed to let in some drying sunlight and give the house a chance to "breathe." Keep the yard free of fallen leaves in autumn.

When painting indoor walls, use a mold-inhibiting paint or add a mold inhibitor to the paint, especially in rooms that are likely to get damp and areas with brick or cinderblock walls. Cement floors in basements and garages should be painted with waterproofing paint. Avoid laying carpeting on a concrete floor; vinyl flooring (sheet type, not tiles) is preferable. If a carpet gets very wet, say, from a leak in the roof or a pipe, and smells of mildew, consider replacing it.

Fix all leaks as soon as possible. If water collects in the crawl space under the house or forms mini-pools near the house, correct the drainage problem. In some cases, this may require installation of one or more drainage pipes to funnel the water away from the house. If there is a dirt surface under the house, install a plastic vapor barrier over the dirt and insulation under the floor of the house to keep moisture from rising up and to reduce condensation on the floorboards.

Avoid using pillows, mattresses, and furniture that are filled with foam rubber; sweat makes them moldy. Choose instead furnishings labeled "hypoallergenic."

If You Use a Humidifier   Many people have problems with humidifiers. They start out with the best of intentions about keeping them clean, but soon tire of the regimen and unintentionally set the stage for an allergic disaster. Though it is logical to want to moisturize heated air, which can become drier than a desert, any container that holds water at room temperature is likely to breed molds. Failure to closely adhere to manufacturers' directions about regular and thorough cleansing of humidifiers can result in worse problems than the ones you are trying to solve. This applies as well to central humidifiers that are installed on the furnace. Humidifiers that get moldy simply spray the allergenic spores into the air you breathe. Some newer humidifiers have been designed to prevent mold growth through a special heating process, although these too need regular cleaning. But ultrasonic humidifiers, which initially had been touted as preventing mold problems, were later shown to be even more effective than older, cheaper humidifiers at distributing allergens in the air.

Personally, I prefer a steam vaporizer, since most molds cannot survive in boiling hot water. But here, too, it is important to wash the device properly before refilling it and not to let it stand around with water in it when it is not operating. Molds will grow in the standing water, and at least one allergenic mold thrives in hot water. Ideally, when using any sort of humidifying device, it would be wise to simultaneously operate a HEPA air filter that would pick up any mold spores that enter the air.

Dust Mites

The mites that live in house dust are perhaps the hardest allergen source to avoid. They are ubiquitous and perennial. Still, there are many measures you can take to reduce your exposure to these pesky allergens.

Throughout the House   Keep things simple, neat, and clean. Avoid decorating with dust collectors. The fewer knick-knacks, the better. Open shelving invites dust. Books and magazines are best stored in closed cupboards. Do not save stacks of newspapers or create piles of papers that sit around for weeks. Keep children's toys in a box with a lid.

On windows, use shades, vertical blinds, or washable curtains that are washed frequently; horizontal blinds and drapes are great dust collectors. If your home is heated by hot air, cover the vents with dust-proof filters that let the heat through but keep dust mites out.

In the Bedroom   Just as you no doubt seek comfort in your bed, so do the resident dust mites. To reduce your exposure to them, encase the mattress, box spring, and pillows in zippered, dust-proof covers. Avoid pillows and comforters filled with feathers; dust mites find them even more comfortable than you do. Also avoid using blankets and quilts that require dry cleaning or that would be damaged by hot water. Wash sheets, pillowcases, mattress pad, and blankets every two weeks in hot water (130°F). If you use a comforter that is not encased in an allergen-proof cover, wash it as well. A recent study in Japan showed that while dry cleaning blankets reduced dust-mite allergens by 70 percent, a hot-water washing got rid of more than 95 percent of them.

Dust mites also love rugs, carpets, and upholstered furniture. A wood floor or vinyl floor covering is preferable for the bedroom. If you use scatter rugs, make sure they are washable and washed often. If the room is to remain carpeted, consider using benzyl benzoate moist powder—for example, a product called Acarosan—every three months to kill dust mites. The product is sold in pharmacies and must be vacuumed up. However, since it is the dust-mite excrement and not the mite itself that is allergenic, consider also treating your carpets with a 3% tannic acid spray, such as Allergy Control Solution. Tannins denature the proteins in the dust-mite excrement and render them nonallergenic. Studies have shown the tannic acid treatment to be more effective than benzyl benzoate at reducing dust-mite allergen. There is one problem, however; tannic acid may stain light-colored fabrics.

Caution: When carpets are being cleaned and especially when the treatments are being vacuumed up, those with dust-mite allergies are best off staying out of the house.

Substitute wood, leather, vinyl, plastic, or cloth bedroom furnishings for upholstered ones. Avoid hard-to-clean wall hangings, like pennants and macramé, and stuffed animals unless they are washable and washed often (Gund makes washable stuffed animals). Don't use the bedroom to store books, toys, and other dust collectors.

Closets are notoriously dusty. Store clothing in another room, if possible, or enclose garments in zippered vinyl garment bags. Keep the closet floor as clear as possible and vacuum it regularly, and keep the closet door closed. Clothes that are put away for the season should be stored in a dry place and laundered or dry-cleaned before they are worn again.

If there is one room in the house that should have a HEPA air filter, it is the bedroom. Be sure to follow the manufacturer's recommendation for replacing the machine's activated charcoal filter (usually every three months). The HEPA filter should last three to five years.

House Cleaning   The key words are *often* and *well.* Brooms stir up dust; so do ordinary dry dust cloths. And the exhaust from vacuums sends dust clouds and mites into the air. You can buy a special allergy-control vacuum cleaner; one brand uses multilayer dust bags, another is equipped with a HEPA filter and microfilter on the motor. Or you can adapt your regular vacuum cleaner to reduce the amount of allergens that escape by using a multilayer bag and adding an electrostatically charged exhaust filter.

Dust twice a week with a damp cloth or use dust cloths and mop covers that have been specially treated to attract dust and diminish scatter. They can be washed many times before they lose this property.

If you have a dust-mite allergy, wear a mask when cleaning, such as the 3M Dust and Pollen Filter Mask available in most hardware stores and pharmacies.

When Traveling   If you will be staying at a hotel, motel, or guest house, call before you arrive to request that special care be taken in dusting and vacuuming your room. Ask that synthetic pillows and blankets be placed on the bed or consider bringing along your own bedding, especially if you are sensitive to the harsh detergents commonly used by hotel laundries.

When making your reservation and again when you are checking in, ask for a no-smoking room; these rooms are now widely available in larger hotels and chains.

If you are sensitive to the scents used in many soaps, shampoos, conditioners, and body lotions, be sure to bring along your own.

If your host has decorated your room with a vase of flowers, potpourri, or a plant that tickles your nose, discreetly place it in the closet or suggest that it be moved to a common room so that everyone can enjoy it.

ANIMAL DANDER

I left this for last because it is the hardest, emotionally at least. Many people do not discover their allergy to a pet until the animal has captured their heart. In some cases, in fact, the allergy does not develop until a person has had the pet for some time. Unfortunately, the best way to reduce exposure to allergens from pets is to get rid of the pet that is the source of the problem. Easier said than done! Losing a household pet is like losing a much-loved member of the family. Failing that option, there are others that might help.

Choose Pets Wisely   If any member of the family is known to have nasal allergies, select a pet that does not have fur or feathers. You may think the person is allergic just to cats, only to discover after a newly acquired puppy has won everyone's heart that the person is also allergic to dogs. Among safer possibilities are tropical fish, lizards, snakes, turtles, and insects—not exactly cuddly, but they can have their rewards.

In general, dogs are less likely to provoke allergic reactions than cats, possibly because cats are forever licking themselves and depositing allergens on their fur and skin. However, even among cats, there are differences. For example, I am much more sensitive to Siamese cats than to other breeds I've been around. Also, female cats tend to be less allergenic than male cats, and male cats that have been neutered (a good idea in any event) are less allergenic than male cats with their reproductive apparatus intact.

Reduce Exposure   If you already have an allergen-producing pet that a member of the family is allergic to, it had best become an outdoor pet. Keep in mind, though, that even after a cat is completely banished from a home and the home is thoroughly cleaned, it can take three or four months before cat allergen is gone from carpets and furnishings. If you cannot relegate your pet completely to the outdoors, at the very least keep it outside for as much of the 24-hour day as possible, and do not allow it to sit on cloth-covered furniture.

If you are allergic to the pet and are the only one around to care for it, use an allergen-filtering face mask when brushing it or cleaning out its living quarters, always wash your hands after petting it, and change clothes after holding it.

Even if the animal never goes into the room in which the allergic person sleeps, the bedroom air can become contaminated with the animal's allergens through heating vents. If the animal is in the house at all, make sure the vents are covered with allergen-proof filters. Or, in the allergic person's bedroom, you can close the vent and use an electric heater instead.

Consider also using a HEPA air cleaner, which can reduce the amount of airborne cat allergen by about 50 percent. Since cat allergens stick to clothing, they can also be carried from room to room by someone who handles the animal. Use a vacuum fitted with a HEPA filter; a multilayer dust bag and exhaust filter are often not adequate to control cat allergen, which is very, very tiny.

Wash the Cat   Most cats are notorious for their dislike of water. "I'll clean myself, thank you very much," they seem to say. But since it is just this cleaning—with cat saliva—that is responsible for allergic reactions, it is much better to wash the cat yourself on a regular basis to reduce the amount of salivary allergen it spreads around.

Kittens usually do not mind being washed, so if you are starting out with a kitten, get it used to having a bath every two or three weeks. A mature cat is another story; it has to be gradually "conditioned" to being bathed. Start out by bringing the cat near the sink (or wherever it will be washed), turn on the water, and give the cat a treat or feed it. The next day, turn on the water, wet your hand or a cloth and place it on the cat, and give your pet another treat or feeding. Day by day, gradually increase the amount of water you place on the cat, each time supplying a treat or feeding, until the cat will tolerate having a pitcher of water poured over it. Once you get to this point, for about three weeks wash the cat each week, then at intervals of two to three weeks. The cat should continue to tolerate the bath, but don't expect any thanks.

After all that, you may be disappointed to learn that even with a well-washed cat in the house, a fair amount of cat allergen will continue to float in the air, so consider also using a HEPA air filter (and HEPA vacuum). If you've done everything you can to reduce exposure and cat allergy symptoms still occur but you are unwilling or unable to part with the cat, consider immunotherapy (allergy shots) to reduce your sensitivity—see pages 109–12.

PREVENTING ALLERGIES IN YOUR UNBORN CHILD

When a mother or father has allergies, and especially when both do, their children are at increased risk of also developing allergies. But various studies have strongly suggested that measures taken during pregnancy and after the baby is born can significantly reduce the child's risk of developing allergic rhinitis and other allergic manifestations, such as skin allergies. Even what you feed the baby can make a big difference.

According to Dr. Yalamanchi K. Rao, an allergist affiliated with New York Methodist Hospital in Brooklyn, New York, here are some steps you and your spouse can take to protect your future children if either or both of you are allergic.

- During pregnancy, avoid drinking too much cow's milk or eating many eggs or peanuts. Studies conducted at the University of Saskatchewan showed that umbilical-cord blood of babies born to allergic parents already had high levels of IgE antibodies to milk, eggs, and peanuts if the mother consumed much of these foods during pregnancy. Instead of milk, eat ample amounts of calcium-rich vegetables (collards, kale, etc.) and take a calcium supplement to meet your increased need for calcium during pregnancy.

- After delivery, feed the baby only breast milk for at least six months. If this is not possible, a hypoallergenic alternative is a formula called Good Start made by Carnation. But avoid soy milk; it is as likely as cow's milk and cow's milk formulas to provoke allergies.

- When breast-feeding, it is also helpful for the mother to

avoid consuming common allergenic foods: cow's milk, eggs, peanuts, and wheat products.

- Do not allow any smoking in the house or in any vehicle the baby habitually rides in. That means no smoking in the bathroom or basement either, since the tobacco pollutants readily permeate the air throughout a home no matter where in the dwelling they originate—and even if you cannot smell them elsewhere.
- Reduce the baby's exposure to dust mites by enclosing the crib mattress in a zippered, allergen-proof cover. Use only washable bedding and wash the baby's bedding often in hot (130°F) water. Allow no furry or feathered pets in the room and no stuffed animals (except, perhaps, those by Gund, which are washable—and be sure to wash them often). Use shades or vertical blinds on the windows and wood or vinyl covering on the floor.
- Keep no cats or dogs in the house. No matter where pets spend their days and nights, allergens from animals can permeate a household in the same way tobacco smoke does. Also, adults who regularly care for the baby should avoid handling allergenic pets, since caretakers' clothing and skin will carry the animal's allergens to the baby.
- Do not introduce any solid foods until after the baby is six months old. Start with rice cereal prepared with water; it is the least allergenic. Avoid mixed cereals made with milk. Introduce vegetables before fruits; they are less allergenic and, by not starting the baby off on sweet-tasting fruit, you will increase the chances that the baby will like vegetables.
- Do not give the baby egg white in any form until one year of age. The yolk is okay *if the egg is first hard-boiled* and then the yolk is removed, free of any white. Check ingredients labels on all prepared foods since many products—such as cookies and ice cream—are made with whole eggs or egg whites.

- To reduce the risk of skin allergies (eczema and itchy skin), which are often a prelude to nasal allergies, use a mild cleansing bar (not soap) like Dove or Oil of Olay to wash the baby. Dress the baby in cotton clothing, wash the baby's clothes in a mild, unscented detergent like Arm & Hammer, and rinse the baby's clothes twice to get rid of any detergent residue.

CHECKLIST: Control Your Exposure to Allergens

Controlling allergens in the places where you spend most of your time—your home, your car, and on your job—is the most important step in preventing allergic reactions. Even a squeaky clean house can be full of allergens lurking in unsuspected places. Also important is avoiding irritants that can aggravate an allergic reaction. Here is a quick checklist to help you reduce your exposure to allergens and the symptoms that can result.

At Home

❑ **Use shades or vertical blinds and washable curtains** instead of horizontal blinds and drapes.

❑ **Avoid feather and wool bedding.** Replace feather pillows and down comforters with polyester-filled (hypoallergenic) items and buy new pillows every year. Use washable blankets and quilts and wash them often.

❑ **Avoid dust-catching clutter.** Use enclosed places to keep books, toys, and clothing and keep the closet doors closed. Keep surfaces free of knickknacks.

❑ **Keep floors bare or use washable throw rugs** instead of area rugs and carpets.

❑ **Dry wet clothing immediately,** preferably in a clothes dryer that is vented to the outside.

❑ **Periodically check stored food** in the refrigerator and cupboard and discard anything that shows signs of spoilage or mold. Clean up spills immediately.

❏ **Put filters over forced-air heating vents** and change the filters regularly.

❏ **Install exhaust fans** in the bathroom and over the stove to remove excess moisture and irritating cooking odors.

❏ **Buy one or more air purifiers**—the HEPA kind—for your bedroom and any other room in which you spend a lot of time. Be sure to change the filters when the manufacturer says you should.

❏ **Avoid using humidifiers** and, if necessary, buy a dehumidifier to reduce excess moisture in your home.

❏ **Clean the house weekly** with a HEPA vacuum (or ordinary vacuum fitted with a special filter) and with a damp or specially treated dust cloth.

❏ **Keep rain gutters clean** by regularly removing leaves and debris, which can grow mold.

❏ **Correct drainage problems** around your home to reduce moisture and mold growth.

❏ **Avoid yardwork** that increases your exposure to pollen and molds, such as mowing, raking, and weeding. Or wear a pollen-filtering mask when you work in the yard.

❏ **Keep your car clean** by vacuuming the seats and carpets regularly. Use the car air conditioner instead of opening windows during pollen seasons.

At Work

❏ **Keep your work area uncluttered.** Piles of papers attract dust and molds.

❏ **Dust your work area regularly** with a damp or treated cloth.

❏ **Do not decorate your work area with live plants or dried flowers.** They can grow mold and collect dust.

❏ **Use an air purifier**—HEPA type—to clean the air around your work area.

Avoid Irritants

❏ **Ask friends and co-workers not to smoke or use strong scents** when you are around. They can aggravate allergic symptoms. And, of course, don't smoke or wear scents yourself.

❏ **Avoid using powders and aerosol sprays,** which can be very irritating to the nose.

❏ **Use household cleaners, paints, and other volatile substances only in well-ventilated areas.** Or get someone else to apply them and leave the house until the odor dissipates.

Is School the Source of Your Child's Allergies?

You may be super-conscientious about controlling your allergic child's exposure to allergens at home, only to have it all undone when the child goes to school. If your child continues to have allergy symptoms despite your efforts, visit the classroom to check for sources of allergens and irritants.

The trip to school.

Retrace the steps your child takes to get to school. Does it take him or her near ragweed or heavily polluted roadways? Are there exposures on the school bus that could be a problem, such as open windows that invite in pollen or a driver drenched in cologne? Is the walkway outside the school polluted with cigarette smoke by parents and teachers who have yet to quit this noxious weed?

In the classroom.

Are furry or feathered pets or lots of plants kept in the classroom? Are there stacks of dusty or moldy papers? Do strong odors emanate from science or art projects? Is the coat closet full of dusty forgotten items? Are pungent cleaning products used in the classroom and/or the restrooms? Does the teacher wear a strong scent?

Class trips and outings.

Is your child's class taken outside to play in or near fields that may be loaded with pollen and molds? Are there visits to places that may harbor lots of airborne allergens? Perhaps the teacher will consider scheduling field trips for times of the year when pollen counts are low. Or the teacher might be willing to choose less troublesome destinations.

Choose medication wisely.

Ask your child's physician to recommend or prescribe allergy medications that won't interfere with school performance, such as nasal steroids or non-sedating antihistamines.

Check the school's policy.

If your child will need to have medication administered during the school day, ask if there is a school nurse to help out. If the medication can be self-administered, tell the teacher the child will be taking medication while in school.

7

TREATING NASAL ALLERGIES

I
f the preventive techniques described in the preceding chapters fail to contain your allergic symptoms enough so that you can live comfortably with your enemy, it's time to bring on the heavy artillery. Among the options are these:

- Cromolyn sodium nasal spray, which blocks the inflammatory response to airborne allergens and can often nip the allergic reaction in the bud.

- Antihistamines of various kinds, which counter the classic symptoms of allergic rhinitis by blocking the action of histamine, the irritating chemical released in nasal and surrounding tissues when you inhale an allergen.

- Decongestants to relieve nasal and sinus congestion.

- Nasal rinses and eye drops to soothe irritated tissues.

- Corticosteroid nasal sprays, which reduce the inflammation in the nasal passages that results in a runny or stuffy nose, sneezing, and nasal itching.

- Immunotherapy (allergy shots) to suppress your body's tendency to treat innocent substances like pollen grains and mold spores as archenemies.

Everyone with allergic rhinitis should be helped by one or more of these regimens *if the treatment program is followed as prescribed.* Just as it may do you no good to take an antibiotic for three days when it was prescribed for ten, you are unlikely to get the allergy relief you seek if you repeatedly start and stop allergy shots or wait until your symptoms have become intolerable before you take antihistamines.

ANTIHISTAMINES, THE ENEMY OF ALLERGIES

Even people without allergies know about antihistamines, and more than 30 million Americans with allergies take them every year. Antihistamines are among the most widely advertised "consumer" drugs, and are often misused by people with colds (antihistamines are common—albeit inappropriate—ingredients in over-the-counter cold and flu "remedies"). However, they are highly effective in countering allergic reactions. Various studies have shown that up to 85 percent of people with seasonal allergic rhinitis get good to excellent relief from antihistamines.

Perhaps you are wary of antihistamines, having tried them in the past and found that it was hard to stay awake and alert. It may be time for you to give these highly effective allergy fighters a second look. In recent years, three new kinds have been introduced that are unlikely to cause grogginess, cloud your concentration, wreck your coordination, or slow your reaction time, and one or another of these new antihistamines has come to spell relief for millions of Americans with allergic rhinitis. They are administered as tablets, and need to be taken only once or twice a day, instead of every four to six hours, to keep symptoms at bay.

You may recall from Chapter 2, "How Allergies Happen," that histamine is the main body chemical that triggers symptoms of nasal allergies. Once released by mast cells, histamines attach themselves to receptors on the walls of nearby blood vessels, ir-rritating them and causing swelling, secretions, and itching. An-tihistamines work just as you might expect: they "coat" the receptors for histamine and prevent it from making its symptom-provoking connections with blood vessel walls. They begin to work about 15 to 30 minutes after they are taken and reach max-imum effectiveness in 1 to 2 hours. They are highly effective in countering immediate, or early-phase, allergic reactions that re-sult in sneezing, itching, and runny nose and they partially re-duce the congestion of allergic rhinitis. However, antihistamines have no effect on the delayed inflammatory reactions to nasal allergens that afflict about half of the people with seasonal al-lergic rhinitis. For such people to get maximum relief, a com-bination of antihistamines and nasal steroids is needed.

As you might guess, antihistamines are most effective if taken *before* you are exposed to the allergen that provokes your symp-toms and if you continue to take them until you are no longer exposed. Say you want to control your allergic reaction to grass or ragweed pollen. To get the most you can from this therapy, you would have to take antihistamines daily for about two months until the offending pollen clears out of the air.

Antihistamines are also an excellent way to squelch the symp-toms of allergic rhinitis that are provoked by occasional expo-sures. For example, I am allergic to cats. I do not have a cat myself, but when I am invited to someone's house who does have a cat, I take an antihistamine about half an hour before I arrive. If I am going to spend one or more nights in a "cat house," I continue to take antihistamines until I get home and out of the clothes I wore that may still be carrying cat allergen. I am also allergic to mold spores, which are readily stirred up when I garden, an avocation I would hate to give up. So before I don my gardening clothes, I pop an antihistamine in my mouth. My husband, who has a sometimes dramatic dust-mite allergy as well as an allergy to mold spores, takes an antihistamine before he starts ferreting around in the basement, stirring up dust and mold that inevitably settle on the items we store there.

Two Kinds of Antihistamines Until about a decade ago, all antihistamines were plagued by a sometimes unfortunate side effect: they could enter the brain and make people tired, sluggish, and sleepy, compounding the effects of the allergy itself. All carried a warning that users should not operate motor vehicles or dangerous machinery. In our automobile-dependent society, this made antihistamines a serious risk for millions of people who might otherwise benefit from their use. Although the sedative effects of antihistamines often wear off after they are taken for a few weeks, most people who need them cannot afford to wait that long to drive again or to work with hazardous equipment.

But since these antihistamines are sold over-the-counter and since many people fail to read labels, there is no way to be sure users will heed the warnings. Highway safety experts say that many fatal accidents are caused by sleepy drivers drugged by medications, including antihistamines. One study showed, for example, that drivers who caused their own fatal accidents were 1.5 times more likely to have taken a sedating antihistamine than those drivers not responsible for their own death. The sedative effects of these drugs are multiplied when the person also consumes even a small amount of alcohol or takes another medication with similar effects on the brain.

Sedating antihistamines can also impair a person's ability to concentrate and do desk work. Some people are highly sensitive to the sedative effects of these drugs; others are not. And all sedating antihistamines are not equally sedating. Brompheniramine (Dimetane), chlorpheniramine (Chlor-Trimeton, Teldrin), cetirizine (Zyrtec), and clemastine (Tavist) are less troublesome than diphenhydramine (Benadryl), promethazine

Table 8: **Common**

Generic Name	Trade Name	How Sold
Sedating:		
Cetirizine	Zyrtec	Rx
Chlorpheniramine	Chlor-Trimeton	OTC
	Teldrin	
Clemastine	Tavist	OTC
		Rx
	Tavist Syrup	Rx
Cyproheptadine	Periactin	Rx
	Periactin Syrup	Rx
Diphenhydramine	Benadryl	OTC
Hydroxyzine	Atarax	Rx
Promethazine	Phenergan	Rx
Tripelennamine	PBZ	Rx
	PBZ-SR	Rx
Non-sedating:		
Astemizole	Hismanal	Rx
Fexofenadine	Allegra	Rx
Loratadine	Claritin	Rx
*Terfenadine	Seldane	Rx

*As of this writing, the Food and Drug Administration had proposed to ban Seldane because of rare but potentially deadly heart rhythm abnormalities when taken with certain antibiotics (see page 87). The same risk applies to Hismanal.

Types of Antihistamines

Dose	How Often Taken
10 mg	Once a day
4 mg	Every 4–6 hours
8 mg	Every 8–12 hours
12 mg	Every 12 hours
12 mg	Every 12 hours
1.34 mg	Every 12 hours
2.68 mg	No more than every 8 hours
0.5 mg	Every 12 hours
4 mg	Every 8 hours
2 mg	Every 8–12 hours
25 to 50 mg	Every 4–6 hours
25, 50, 100 mg	Every 6–8 hours
12.5, 25 mg	Every 4–6 hours
25 to 50 mg	Every 4–6 hours
100 mg	Every 12 hours
10 mg	Once a day
60 mg	Every 12 hours
10 mg	Once a day
60 mg	Every 12 hours

(Phenergan), and tripelennamine (PBZ). Yet in various studies even chlorpheniramine caused sedation in 10 to 25 percent of users.

To provide more effective allergy relief, antihistamines are often sold in combination with decongestants. When the antihistamine has a sedating effect, the combination is fortuitous; since decongestants act as stimulants of the central nervous system (see page 88), they help to counter the sleep-inducing effects of these antihistamines.

Now, however, there are other options. Pharmaceutical chemists have designed antihistamines that cannot readily cross from the blood into the brain and therefore only rarely cause drowsiness. Thus far, these drugs are available only by prescription, although sooner or later one or more are likely to be sold over-the-counter. Right now, as prescription drugs, these medications can make a serious dent in your budget if your insurance doesn't cover most or all of their cost. If you have allergies, by now you've probably heard about one or more of these medications, if not through direct advertising then from fellow sufferers who swear by them. There are three kinds of nonsedating antihistamines now marketed: terfenadine (Seldane), loratadine (Claritin), and astemizole (Hismanal). Unlike over-the-counter antihistamines, which have to be taken two to six times daily to get the maximum benefit, these prescription medications are longer-acting and need only be taken once or twice a day.

Warning: Do Not Take Antihistamines If . . .   Unless advised by a physician who is familiar with the patient's medical history and the side effects of the various antihistamines, these drugs should not be taken by nursing mothers, people with obstructions of the bladder or stomach, people with narrow-angle glaucoma or certain types of peptic ulcers, and any patient taking an antidepressant drug called an MAO (monoamine oxidase) inhibitor (Nardil and Parnate, among others).

Phenergan, which is a strong sedative, should not be taken in conjunction with narcotic painkillers, barbiturates, alcohol, or tranquilizers.

Seldane and Hismanal should not be taken by people with liver disease and those who are being treated with any antifungal agents, especially Nizoral (ketoconazole) and Sporanox (itraconazole), or with the antibiotics erythromycin (many brands and generic), Biaxin (clarithromycin), Zithromax (azithromycin), or TOA (troleandomycin). For such patients, the prescription antihistamine Claritin or any of the over-the-counter antihistamines would be a safer choice.

Antihistamines also carry a warning against their use by people with asthma. This is in part to prevent such patients from attempting to treat themselves, which can be very dangerous. The warning also stems from the fact that antihistamines dry out and thicken respiratory secretions and may make it harder for asthma patients to clear their air passages.

DECONGESTANTS: UNSTUFFING THE ALLERGIC HEAD

Decongestants shrink swollen nasal tissues by constricting blood vessels, which reduces blood flow to mucous membranes. This opens up breathing passages and relieves sinus pressure. As with antihistamines, decongestants are sold both over-the-counter and by prescription. They also come in two different formulations: as oral medications and as nasal sprays or drops. Each has its advantages and disadvantages. Nasal sprays and drops act quickly, often within moments, to clear nasal passages. They are excellent for providing temporary relief of nasal congestion and for keeping the ears open when descending in an airplane.

Unfortunately, people can become "addicted" to their nasal spray. If used for more than a week at a time, nasal decongestants can actually cause further congestion as soon as the medication wears off, which happens more and more quickly with continued use. This rebound reaction, called chemical rhinitis or rhinitis medicamentosa (medicine-induced rhinitis), necessitates a very uncomfortable weaning process to restore normal nasal function.

Therefore, oral decongestants are the treatment of choice if treatment of nasal congestion is likely to be needed for more than a few days. Oral decongestants take a lot longer to act. They stimulate the central nervous system, which is fine during the day but may interfere with sound sleep at night. They may also be appetite suppressants. The most widely used oral decongestants, both in over-the-counter and in prescription drugs, are pseudoephedrine (for example, Sudafed and Actifed), phenylpropanolamine (for example, Propagest, Rhindecon, and Entax), and phenylephrine (mainly in combination prescription products). As an appetite suppressant, phenylpropanolamine, or PPA, is the active ingredient in over-the-counter diet pills.

Cautions   Oral decongestants should be used with caution by people with enlarged prostates, diabetes, or overactive thyroids. Because decongestants act by constricting blood vessels, they raise blood pressure and heart rate and can be a hazard to people with cardiovascular problems. Persons with high blood pressure or any kind of heart problem and those taking betablockers (Inderal, Lopressor, and Tinormin, among others) or the anti-Parkinson's drug methyldopa should consult a physician before using an oral decongestant. Nursing mothers should not take phenylpropanolamine. In general, women who are pregnant or nursing should always consult their physicians before taking any medications.

TOPICAL NASAL SPRAYS

For many people, the best way to control allergy symptoms is at their source: the nose. They may be unable to take oral medications that can affect other bodily functions or that may interact with other medications they must take. Or they may prefer not to subject their whole bodies and brains to a drug effect when what is really needed is some local action. For them, topical treatments applied directly to the nose may be the answer. Although topical decongestants (nasal sprays and drops) cannot safely be used long-term (see page 88), the medications described below can provide safe and effective symptom relief throughout the allergy season and even year-round. Their main disadvantage is their inability to fully counter allergy symptoms in the eyes and mouth; those bothered by itchy, red eyes or an itchy palate may also have to take an antihistamine to obtain more complete relief.

Cromolyn Sodium, a Safe Symptom Stopper   Cromolyn sodium nasal spray, marketed as Nasalcrom, is perhaps the most underappreciated and underutilized remedy for nasal allergies. It is a highly effective nonsteroidal drug that can stop nasal allergic reactions before they start, countering both immediate and delayed symptoms. It has been shown to relieve nasal itching, sneezing, runny nose, and congestion in people with allergic rhinitis. It appears to work by stabilizing the mast cells and preventing them from releasing histamine and other symptom-causing chemicals.

Cromolyn sodium is most effective if its use is begun before the start of the allergy season and it is continued until you are no longer exposed to the offending allergen(s). It is now sold without a prescription. Nonetheless, this therapy is extremely safe, even for those who may be unable to use other treatments to control their symptoms. It can be used safely by children, the elderly, pregnant women, and people who are taking medications that may interfere with other allergy-fighting drugs. Because it is given topically rather than by mouth or injection, it has no effects elsewhere in the body—only in the nose. Its rare side effects may include sneezing, a burning sensation in the nose, nasal irritation, and headache. What is more, it will not cause the rebound congestion that results from prolonged use of nasal decongestants. All told, cromolyn sodium has the fewest side effects of any allergy-fighting medication.

So why don't more people with allergies know about and use it? Allergists say it is primarily because patients have to apply the nasal spray about four to six times a day to reap the full benefit of the medication, and most Americans simply can't be bothered. They'd rather pop a pill or two and take a chance on side effects than administer a nasal spray four times a day.

Corticosteroid Nasal Sprays, Also Safe and Underused
Many Americans hear the words "cortisone" and "steroid" and panic. They immediately recall warnings that corticosteroids administered by mouth or injection can shut down the body's own production of adrenal hormones, cause bloating and weight gain, or otherwise disrupt bodily functions. But when applied only to the nose, as with anti-allergy corticosteroid sprays, the steroidal effect is local and the adrenal glands continue to function normally even if the nasal spray is used all year long.

Nasal corticosteroid sprays are the most potent medications available for treating allergic rhinitis. Products, all of which are available only with a doctor's prescription, include beclomethasone (Beconase and Vancenase), budesonide (Rhinocort), flunisolide (Nasaral), fluticasone propionate (Flonase), and triamcinolone acetonide (Nasacort). As with cromolyn sodium, corticosteroid sprays work best when used in advance of an allergic attack, starting a week or so prior to exposure to the offending allergen. Once you have symptoms, the response to treatment is likely to be slow.

Corticosteroid sprays have potent anti-inflammatory effects on nasal membranes and, like cromolyn sodium, inhibit both immediate and delayed allergic reactions. They are more effective than cromolyn at quelling allergic symptoms and are especially effective against the delayed reactions. They also reduce nasal sensitivity to irritants like smoke and strong scents, and they reduce, though they may not entirely eliminate, itching in the eyes and mouth.

A further advantage of these products is that they need only be used once or twice a day. They can be used safely and effectively both for seasonal and perennial allergic rhinitis.

The main disadvantages of nasal corticosteroids include possible irritation of the nasal lining, a delayed response to treatment, failure to completely control eye symptoms, and the need for physicians to check patients periodically for possible nasal problems, a rare consequence of prolonged use. Although most of the medications in this category have been approved for use by children over age six, few are available for use in younger children.

Atrovent, New Kid on the Block   Of much more limited usefulness is ipratropium bromide (Atrovent), recently approved for use as a nasal spray. It is a drying agent that is excellent at countering a runny nose but has no effect on sneezing, itching, or nasal congestion. It is in a class of drugs called anticholinergics and can sometimes cause excessive nasal dryness.

Saline Nasal Sprays   Saline, or salt water, is often used as a non-therapeutic, or inactive, agent in testing the value of other products. Here, though, it shines on its own. Saline nasal sprays are especially useful in relieving nasal stuffiness, sneezing, and congestion in people with perennial rhinitis. And they are perfectly safe for everyone, no matter how long or how often they are used.

Two similar products, propylene and polyethylene glycol nasal sprays, are equally safe and effective. As "wetting agents" that temporarily coat the nasal membranes, these nasal sprays can help prevent nasal irritation if they are used immediately before applying a corticosteroid nasal spray.

You can easily make your own saline nose drops. Simply add 1/4 teaspoon of ordinary table salt and 1/4 teaspoon of baking soda to 8 ounces of room-temperature water and apply the solution with a bulb syringe or dropper. Or you can buy a ready-made spray or saline nose drops in the drugstore. Popular brands include Ocean, NaSal, and Salinex.

WHEN YOUR EYES ARE RED AND ITCHY

I know this will sound like advice from your mother, but the most important control measure is to stop rubbing your eyes. Rubbing can deposit more allergen into your eyes and may add further to your misery by mechanically causing mast cells on the surface of the eye and in the lid to discharge their load of histamines. Sometimes a cool compress and the use of artificial tears (these have no drug effect but are effective lubricants) can reduce your ocular discomfort sufficiently. Artificial tears contain a demulcent, a substance that coats and protects mucous membranes, helping them to retain moisture and insulating them against environmental insults. You may also wash your eyes as often as you like with a sterile eye-irrigating solution such as the over-the-counter product Dacriose. This kind of eye wash, which has no drug effect and no side effects, may be all you need to control eye irritation caused by nasal allergies.

If medication is needed, cromolyn sodium has been incorporated in eye drops that can reduce the annoying ocular symptoms associated with allergic rhinitis. The product, Cromolon, is available only by prescription. It works as a preventive, keeping the mast cells from releasing histamine. As with cromolyn sodium nasal spray, the eye drops are safe, safer than using oral antihistamines. Unlike steroid eye medications, they do not cause glaucoma or cataracts. The drops can be used four to six times a day. Another product with the same action is Iodoxamide, sold as Alomide, also a prescription drug.

Antihistamines have also been incorporated into prescription eye drops. The product, levocabastine (Livostin), relieves all ocular signs and symptoms of allergic rhinitis. But if itching is your only problem, Acular eye drops containing the nonsteroidal anti-inflammatory drug ketorolac may be all you need to get relief.

There are also various over-the-counter products—for example, Vasocon-A and Naphacon-A—that can provide symptomatic relief. These contain antihistamines, which counter itching and tearing, and low doses of blood-vessel constrictors, which reduce redness. While these products are generally safe, eyes drops that "get the red out" should not be used by people with narrow-angle glaucoma because they can cause partial or total blindness. Nor should anyone use them habitually; constant use of blood-vessel constrictors dries out the eyes and can result in a rebound reaction, causing the eyes to get red as soon as you stop using the drops. So save this remedy for when you really need it. Before you buy eye drops, be sure to check the label for ingredients that are blood-vessel constrictors: naphazoline, ephedrine, phenylephrine, and tetrahydrozoline.

TREATING SPECIAL PEOPLE

How your nasal allergies are best managed often depends upon who you are. Those in need of special consideration include children, pregnant women, athletes, the elderly, and people with certain chronic ailments or those taking certain medications for other health problems (see page 88).

Children   It is important to treat children's allergies aggressively lest they compromise intellectual, academic, and social development and result in serious medical complications. Persistent nasal congestion in infants can result in an accumulation of fluid in the middle ear and repeated ear infections. If not promptly and adequately corrected, these ear problems can interfere with hearing and speech development at a crucial time in the child's life and leave a lifelong legacy.

Allergic rhinitis, which afflicts one in ten school-age children and 20 to 30 percent of adolescents, can interfere with learning and cause irritability, anger, difficulty concentrating, and poor school performance. Indeed, some children with allergic rhinitis are mistakenly labeled "hyperactive" and the true cause of their aberrant behavior is overlooked and untreated. Also, failure to recognize and properly control allergic rhinitis can cause far worse health problems, like asthma and chronic ear infections. Yet proper treatment of childhood allergies can eradicate most if not all of these problems and allow allergic children to achieve their full potential.

Currently the antihistamines approved for use in children under age twelve are all sedating and can interfere with concentration and alertness, with a negative effect on learning and school performance. This is only one reason why the most important step in controlling allergies in the young is to reduce the child's exposure to as many sources of allergens and nasal irritants as possible, especially dust, molds, pets, and tobacco smoke (see pages 65–78). If the child needs medication to control symptoms triggered by unavoidable allergens, the most important thing to remember is that a child is not a small adult. The choice of drugs and the dose must be adjusted not only to the child's weight but also with regard to age, metabolic development, and social needs.

Ideally, children under age six should be treated by a physician trained in pediatric allergy. Few allergy-fighting medications have been approved for use in such young children, and it requires special expertise to choose the right drugs and the right dosages for such youngsters.

For school-age children, experts caution against using oral corticosteroids and nasal decongestant sprays or drops, as well as sedating antihistamines that could interfere with school performance. Unfortunately, the non-sedating antihistamines have been approved only for use in children age twelve and older. However, many allergists will prescribe one or the other of these drugs for younger children at a reduced dose. Experts suggest giving an adult dose to children who weigh more than 62 pounds and cutting the dose for smaller children.

If possible, treatment is best started before the onset of allergy season using nasal cromolyn sodium (Nasalcrom) or, if stronger medication is needed, one of the nasal corticosteroid sprays. Vancenase and Beconase (beclomethasone), which rarely cause side effects, are approved for use in children as young as age six. If a decongestant is needed, pseudoephedrine (Sudafed and its generic mimics) is preferred, up to a daily dose of 60 milligrams. Also helpful, and completely safe, are nasal saline sprays or drops to relieve congestion and irritation.

If the child's symptoms are not adequately controlled through avoidance and medication, immunotherapy—a series of allergy shots—is strongly recommended for children age three and older. Although these shots do not bring immediate relief, if properly administered they can greatly benefit the child's long-term well-being (see pages 109–12).

Pregnant Women Here you have more than the patient to worry about, because any treatment given to a pregnant woman has the potential to affect her unborn child. Thus, topical remedies—nasal cromolyn sodium and nasal saline sprays—are much preferred. Unfortunately, the safety of nasal corticosteroids in pregnancy has not been established, although animal studies have not shown them to cause birth defects. Accordingly, experts say that when considering such treatments during pregnancy, the benefits versus the risks should be carefully weighed.

As for antihistamines, the safety of astemizole (Hismanal) and terfenadine (Seldane) during pregnancy has not been established. However, tripelennamine (PBZ, PBZ-SR) and chlorpheniramine (Chlor-Trimeton and Teldrin), both of which are sedating, and loratadine (Claritin), which is non-sedating, can be used with caution in pregnancy. No risk of birth defects has been seen in animal studies with loratadine, although it has not been tested in people. Tripelennamine and chlorpheniramine have never been scientifically tested for safety in pregnancy because they were approved long before tests during pregnancy were required. However, in a review of drugs taken during pregnancy by thousands of women, no association with birth defects was found in the course of years of clinical experience with tripelennamine and chlorpheniramine.

The decongestant pseudoephedrine (Sudafed) is approved for use in pregnancy, but be sure not to exceed the recommended dosage. To help relieve nasal congestion, especially during sleep, a little Band-Aid-like device called BreatheRight, which fits over the outside of the nose, is often helpful and completely safe.

If a woman is in the midst of immunotherapy when she becomes pregnant, there is no need to stop. But experts suggest that the dose of allergen should not be increased until after childbirth. They also caution against starting a course of immunotherapy during pregnancy.

Athletes   Have you ever noticed that physical exercise "clears the head," not just of bothersome thoughts and emotional stress, but also of congestion? For those who exercise moderately, this beneficial effect often lasts for an hour or so after the activity is stopped. However, after an initial period of decongestion, endurance athletes like long-distance runners and cyclists may experience a persistent rebound reaction that leaves

them congested for hours and may impair their athletic performance. Since many athletic endeavors take place in the "great
outdoors" where airborne allergens abound, athletes may find
it hard to avoid being exposed to the sources of their misery.

In treating competitive athletes, care must be taken not only
to avoid interfering with athletic performance with such treatments as sedating antihistamines, but also to avoid medications
that have "doping properties" or are banned in competitive
sports, such as oral decongestants and corticosteroids. Thus, the
preferred remedies for athletes are non-sedating antihistamines
and nasal corticosteroids (the latter are allowed if the athlete sub-
mits a letter from the prescribing physician describing the need
for the treatment). Better yet, an athlete who prefers not to be
dependent on medication might consider immunotherapy as a
long-term solution (see pages 109–12).

The Elderly   Older people metabolize drugs more slowly,
they are more susceptible to the hazards of sedation, and they
often have other health problems or are taking medications that
can interfere with allergy treatments. As people age, they tend
to become more sensitive to both the sedating and the stimulating effects of medications. As a result, elderly patients may require lower doses of allergy-fighting drugs.

Sedating antihistamines should be avoided in the elderly, who
may experience drug-induced visual difficulties and balance
problems that increase their risk of falls and fractures. Elderly
men may also develop urinary retention on these medications.

Oral decongestants (pseudoephedrine, phenylpropanolamine,
and phenylephrine) should also be avoided, especially in people with high blood pressure, coronary artery disease, glaucoma,
diabetes, and enlarged prostates.

Probably the best treatment for allergic rhinitis in the elderly
is a non-sedating antihistamine, assuming a medication can be
selected that does not interfere with other drugs the person is

taking (see page 88), and/or treatment with nasal cromolyn sodium or nasal corticosteroids.

Table 9: What Drugs Help Which Symptoms?

Drug treatment of allergic rhinitis is likely to bring the best relief if the medication chosen is effective against the patient's most bothersome symptoms. As you can see from this table, most effective in countering classic symptoms of allergic rhinitis are nasal corticosteroids and oral drugs that combine an antihistamine and a decongestant.

Agent	Itching/ Sneezing	Runny Nose	Nasal Blockage	Eye Symptoms
Oral antihistamines	+++	++	+−	+++
Nasal corticosteroids	+++	+++	++	+
Oral decongestants	−	+−	+++	−
Oral antihistamine/ decongestant combinations	+++	++	+++	+++
Nasal decongestants*	−	+−	+++	−
Nasal cromolyn sodium	+	+	+−	−
Nasal anticholinergics	−	+++	−	−
Nasal saline sprays/drops	+	−	+	−
Cromolyn sodium eye drops	−	−	−	++
Antihistamine/decongestant eye drops	−	−	−	++

Key:
− = no effect
+ = an effect
++ = more effective
+++ = most effective
+− = product may or may not help this symptom

Use nasal decongestants for no more than 7 consecutive days.

Table 10: **Choosing an Over-the-Counter Allergy Remedy**

If your allergy symptoms are seasonal and not too severe, self-treatment with one or more over-the-counter medications may get you over the rough time without your having to spend time and money on doctor visits. However, the sheer number of products now on the market—and the fierce competition for the consumer dollar—can end up confusing you more than enlightening you about the relative merits of the various products.

The general rule of therapeutics is simple: determine which of your symptoms is most bothersome and select one or more medications that will counter them. In every case, the simpler the medication, the better. Products with four or five different ingredients are likely to contain doses of the individual ingredients that are too low to be meaningful. Plus, you'll probably end up taking medications you really don't need, which is never a good idea. If you're sneezing and have a runny nose and itchy eyes, you need only an antihistamine, not an analgesic for a nonexistent headache or a decongestant for a nose that isn't stuffy or a cough suppressant for a cough you don't have.

Be sure to check the label—all ingredients must be listed—before you buy. Also check the dosing schedule; if you're the type who never remembers to take medication every 4 or 6 hours, perhaps you ought to choose a product that is administered only once or twice a day.

Elixirs, syrups, and other liquid preparations are designed primarily for use by children. The appropriate dose will depend on the child's age or weight. There are no antihistamines approved for use in children under age two. Be sure to check the label for exact dosing recommendations according to the child's age and/or weight. Adults who have difficulty swallowing tablets or capsules may also take these liquid preparations, but they should consider increasing the dose to equal the amount recommended for adults in tablet or capsule versions of the medication.

Warning: Never give a child allergy medications in doses intended for adults without first consulting the child's physician.

The medications listed below represent products and formulations on the market at the end of 1995. Keep in mind that, like food producers, drug manufacturers are forever changing their products—both the ingredients and dosages and dosing schedules—without changing the product name. *So always read the label before you buy,* even if you have been using a product for years, to be sure you are getting what you expect.

Antihistamines
Note: All over-the-counter antihistamines are sedating. Do not operate a motor vehicle or dangerous machinery while taking them.

Product	What's in It?	How Much? How Often?
Benadryl Elixir	12.5 mg diphenhydramine per teaspoon	½–2 teaspoons every 4–6 hours depending on child's age
Benadryl 25	25 mg diphenhydramine per tablet	1 tablet every 4–6 hours
Clor-Trimeton	Each tablet:	1 tablet:
4 Hour Allergy	4 mg chlorpheniramine	Every 4–6 hours
8 Hour Allergy	8 mg chlorpheniramine	Every 8–12 hours
12 Hour Allergy	12 mg chlorpheniramine	Every 12 hours
Dimetane	4 mg brompheniramine per tablet	1 tablet every 6 hours
Sominex*	25 mg diphenhydramine per tablet	2 at bedtime
	50 mg diphenhydramine per capsule	1 at bedtime
Tavist-1	1.34 mg clemastine per tablet	1 tablet every 12 hours

*Sominex is sold as a sleeping potion, thus the recommendation for bedtime dosing. However, its active ingredient is an antihistamine and can be used as such. For example, as with Benadryl 25, one 25-mg Sominex tablet might be taken once every 4 to 6 hours.

Antihistamine/Decongestant Combinations

Note: All over-the-counter antihistamines are sedating, but the decongestants are stimulating and may counteract the sedation.

Product	What's in It?	How Much? How Often?
Actifed Syrup	30 mg pseudoephedrine & 1.25 triprolidine per teaspoon	1–2 teaspoons every 4–6 hours depending on age
Actifed	60 mg pseudoephedrine & 2.5 mg triprolidine per tablet	½–1 tablet every 4–6 hours depending on age
Actifed Allergy Daytime/ Nightime	*Daytime, each caplet: 30 mg pseudoephedrine Nightime, each caplet: 25 mg diphenhydramine 30 mg pseudoephedrine	2 caplets every 4–6 hours 2 caplets at bedtime
Allerest Maximum Strength	2 mg chlorpheniramine & 30 mg pseudoephedrine per tablet	2 tablets every 4–6 hours
Allerest 12 Hour Caplets	12 mg chlorpheniramine & 75 mg phenylpropanolamine per caplet	1 caplet every 12 hours
Allerest Children's Chewable Tablets	1 mg chlorpheniramine & 9.4 mg phenylpropanolamine per tablet	2 tablets every 4–6 hours for children 6–12
Benadryl Decongestant Elixir	12.5 mg diphenhydramine & 30 mg pseudoephedrine per teaspoon	½–2 teaspoons every 4–6 hours depending on age
Benadryl Decongestant Tablets	25 mg diphenhydramine & 60 mg pseudoephedrine per tablet	1 tablet every 4–6 hours

Product	What's in It?	How Much? How Often?
Children's Vicks Dayquil Allergy Relief	2 mg chlorpheniramine & 30 mg pseudoephedrine per tablespoon	1 teaspoon–2 tablespoons 4 times a day depending on age
Chlor-Trimeton 4-Hour Allergy/ Decongestant	4 mg chlorpheniramine & 60 mg pseudoephedrine per tablet	1 tablet every 4–6 hours
Chlor-Trimeton 12-Hour Allergy/ Decongestant	8 mg chlorpheniramine & 120 mg pseudoephedrine per tablet	1 tablet every 12 hours
Contac Continuous Action 12 Hour Capsules	8 mg chlorpheniramine & 75 mg phenylpropanolamine per capsule	1 capsule every 12 hours
Contac Maximum Strength 12 Hour Caplets	12 mg chlorpheniramine & 75 mg phenylpropanolamine	1 caplet every 12 hours
Dimetane Decongestant	4 mg chlorpheniramine & 20 mg phenylephrine per tablet	1 tablet every 6 hours
Dimetapp Extentabs	12 mg brompheniramine & 75 mg phenylpropanolamine per tablet	1 tablet every 12 hours
Dimetapp Tablets and Liqui-Gels	4 mg brompheniramine & 25 mg phenylpropanolamine per tablet or gel-cap	1 tablet or gel-cap every 4 hours
Drixoral Cold & Allergy Sustained-Action	6 mg dexbrompheniramine & 120 mg pseudoephedrine per tablet	1 tablet every 12 hours

Product	What's in It?	How Much? How Often?
Novahistine Elixir	2 mg chlorpheniramine & 5 mg phenylephrine per teaspoon	½–2 teaspoons every 4 hours depending on age
Sudafed Plus Liquid	2 mg chlorpheniramine & 30 mg pseudoephedrine per teaspoon	1–2 teaspoons every 4–6 hours depending on age
Sudafed Plus Tablets	4 mg chlorpheniramine & 60 mg pseudoephedrine per tablet	1 tablet every 4–6 hours
Tavist-D	1.34 mg clemastine & 75 mg phenylpropanolamine per tablet	1 tablet every 12 hours
Teldrin 12 Hour	8 mg chlorpheniramine & 75 mg phenylpropanolamine per capsule	1 capsule every 12 hours
Triaminic Allergy Tablets	4 mg chlorpheniramine & 25 mg phenylpropanolamine per tablet	½–1 tablet every 4 hours depending on age
Triaminic Chewables	0.5 chlorpheniramine & 6.25 phenylpropanolamine per tablet	2 tablets every 4 hours
Vicks Dayquil Allergy Relief 4 Hour Tablets	4 mg brompheniramine & 25 mg phenylpropanolamine per tablet	1 tablet every 4 hours
Vicks Dayquil Allergy Relief 12 Hour Extended Release Tablets	12 mg brompheniramine & 75 mg phenylpropanolamine per tablet	1 tablet every 12 hours

Note: Actifed Allergy Daytime Caplets contain only an oral decongestant and may cause nervousness, insomnia, and loss of appetite.

Oral Decongestants
Note: All oral decongestants are stimulating and may cause nervousness, insomnia, and loss of appetite.

Product	What's in It?	How Much? How Often?
Drixoral Non-Drowsy Formula	120 mg pseudoephedrine per tablet	1 tablet every 12 hours
Children's Sudafed	30 mg pseudoephedrine per teaspoon	½–1 teaspoon every 4–6 hours depending on age
Sudafed	30 mg pseudoephedrine per tablet	1–2 tablets every 4–6 hours depending on age
	60 mg pseudoephedrine per talbet	1 tablet every 4–6 hours

Decongestant Nasal Sprays
Warning: Use these products for only 3 days at a time to avoid rebound reaction.

Afrin	0.05% oxymetazoline	2–3 sprays or drops each nostril every 12 hours
Dristan Fast Acting	0.5% phenylephrine & 0.2% pheniramine	1–2 sprays each nostril no more than once every 4 hours
Dristan Long Acting	0.05% oxymetazoline	1–2 sprays each nostril every 12 hours

Product	What's in It?	How Much? How Often?
4-Way Fast Acting	0.5% phenylephrine, 0.2% pyrilamine, & 0.05% naphazoline	2 sprays each nos- no more than once every 4 hours
4-Way Long Lasting	0.05% oxymetazoline	2–3 sprays each nostril no more than once every 10–12 hours
NTZ Long Acting	0.05% oxymetazoline	2–3 sprays or drops each nostril every 12 hours
Neo-Synephrine Pediatric Mild Regular Extra Strength	0.125% phenylephrine 0.25% phenylephrine 0.5% phenylephrine 1.0% phenylephrine	2–3 sprays each nostril no more than once every 4 hours
Neo-Synephrine Maximum Strength 12 Hour	0.05% oxymetazoline	2–3 sprays each nostril no more than once every 10–12 hours
Nostril 1/4% 1/2%	0.25% phenylephrine 0.5% phenylephrine	2–3 sprays each nostril no more than once every 4 hours
Nostrilla Long Acting	0.05% oxymetazoline	2–3 sprays each nostril no more than once every 10–12 hours
Otrivin	0.1% xylometazoline	2–3 sprays or drops each nostril every 8–10 hours

Product	What's in It?	How Much? How Often?
Otrivin Pediatric	0.05% xylometazoline	2–3 drops each nostril every 8–10 hours
Privine	0.05% naphazoline	1–2 sprays or drops each nostril no more than once every 6 hours
Vicks Sinex Regular	0.5% phenylephrine	2–3 sprays each nostril no more than once every 4 hours
Vicks Sinex Long Acting	0.05% oxymetazoline	2–3 sprays each nostril no more than once every 10–12 hours
Vicks Vapor Inhaler	50 mg *l*-desoxyephedrine	1 inhalation each nostril no more than once every 2 hours
Vicks Vatronol	0.5% ephedrine	1 dropper (up to appropriate mark) no more than once every 4 hours

Saline Nasal Sprays and Drops

Ayr Saline	0.65% sodium chloride	Adults: 2 sprays each nostril as needed Children: 2–4 drops every 2 hours as needed

Product	What's in It?	How Much? How Often?
Ocean Mist	0.65% sodium chloride	2 sprays each nostril as needed
NaSal	0.65% sodium chloride	2 sprays or 4–6 drops each nostril as needed
Salinex	0.4% sodium chloride	2 sprays or drops each nostril as needed

Vasoconstricting Eye Drops
Caution: These products relieve redness in the eyes by constricting blood vessels. Constant use may dry the eyes and result in a rebound reaction.

Clear Eyes	0.012% naphazoline & 0.2% glycerin	1–2 drops each eye no more than 4 times daily
Clear Eyes ACR	0.012% naphazoline, 0.25% zinc sulfate, & 0.2% glycerin	1–2 drops each eye no more than 4 times daily
Collyrium Fresh	0.05% tetrahydrozoline & 1.0% glycerin	1–2 drops each eye no more than 4 times daily
Murine Plus	0.5% polyvinyl alcohol, 0.6% povidone, & 0.05% tetrahydrozoline	1–2 drops each eye no more than 4 times daily
Visine L.R.	0.025% oxymetazoline	1–2 drops each eye every 6 hours

Product	What's in It?	How Much? How Often?
Visine Maximum Strength Allergy Releif	0.05% tetrahydrozoline & 0.25% zinc sulfate	1–2 drops each eye no more than 4 times daily
Visine Moisturizing	0.05% tetrahydrozoline & 1.0% polyethylene glycol	1–2 drops each eye no more than 4 times daily
Visine Original	0.05% tetrahydrozoline	1–2 drops each eye no more than 4 times daily

Antihistamine Eye Drops
Note: There are many different brands of over-the-counter eye drops that contain both an antihistamine and a blood-vessel constrictor (to reduce redness). The following are two of the leading products. See caution above for vasoconstricting eye drops.

Vasocon-A	0.05% naphazoline & 0.5% antazoline	1–2 drops each eye every 2–4 hours, no more than 4 times daily
Naphcon-A	0.025% naphazoline & 0.3% pheniramine	1–2 drops each eye every 3–4 hours, no more than 4 times daily

Allergy Shots Can Really Help

Although allergies can't be cured in the true sense of the word, desensitization—a series of injections over a period of months or years—comes closer than anything else to preventing allergic reactions when exposure to the offending allergen cannot be avoided, or when avoidance tactics and allergy-fighting medications are not enough to keep you from experiencing allergic symptoms that disrupt your life. Desensitization is also generally advisable for patients with extreme reactions to inhaled allergens, such as swelling of the face or respiratory distress.

Allergists will usually suggest trying a year of conservative therapy (avoidance and medication) before launching into a series of desensitizing injections, since the shots involve a considerable investment of money and time.

However, when properly done, the injections are highly effective, ultimately protecting about 85 percent of patients against debilitating reactions to inhaled allergens. Allergy shots are the only way to obtain long-lasting protection against substances you cannot avoid and that result in misery for more than a few weeks a year.

Unfortunately, allergy-suppressing shots are not available for all inhaled allergens, and for some, such as tree pollen, only clinical reports attest to the value of desensitization. Careful studies proving its effectiveness against tree pollen have yet to be done.

Desensitization offers the best protection if you happen to be allergic to grass pollen, ragweed, dust mites, cat allergen, and/or the mold *Alternaria*. But even if you have other allergies that currently cannot be battled with shots, controlling those that are amenable to desensitization will often result in diminished reactions to allergens to which you are still sensitive.

But beware of unscrupulous or incompetent physicians who are too quick to offer allergy shots, having recommended them after an inadequate diagnosis based on one or two skin tests and such diffuse symptoms as fatigue, migraine, and depression as well as the more classic signs of allergy like runny nose, itchy eyes and throat, and sinus congestion (see the section on diagnosis, pages 27–30). Be sure you know what you are allergic to and how sensitive you are to various allergens before launching into a desensitization series. Dr. Peter Kohler, of the University of Colorado Medical Center, says that too often "allergy is a waste-basket diagnosis" in which all kinds of symptoms are blamed on allergies to all sorts of substances.

Warning: Allergy shots should be given only by physicians specially trained in allergy and who have emergency resuscitative equipment on hand and know how to use it, for those extremely rare cases in which a patient develops a potentially life-threatening adverse reaction to an injection of allergens.

How the Shots Work   Allergy shots are a little like the proverbial "hair of the dog." You are given gradually increasing doses of the very substances you are allergic to until your body can tolerate exposure to real-life allergens without reacting to them. Desensitization is something like sibling rivalry. It is a form of immunotherapy in which one arm of the immune system is marshaled to protect against another arm responsible for the immune error that results in the allergic response.

When a patient is injected with tiny doses of the allergen—doses so small they cause no allergic symptoms—the body produces protective "blocking" antibodies called IgG. IgG antibodies, which circulate in the blood, combine with the allergen before it can get to the allergen-specific IgE antibodies that are sitting on mast cells. By preventing a hookup between IgE and the allergen it recognizes, the IgG–allergen union blocks the release of histamine from mast cells. The shots also help to reduce the production of troublesome IgE antibodies. Gradually, over a period of years, the allergen-specific IgE antibodies die off and, as long as there are blocking IgG antibodies present, they will not reform. Or, even if some are manufactured, they are unlikely to reach a level that causes significant symptoms.

If the therapy is done properly, within four to six months a dose is reached that approximates the patient's exposure to the allergen in the course of daily living. Then a maintenance dose must be given for several years to adequately suppress the allergic response.

Desensitization occurs most quickly if the patient is allergic to only one or two substances—say, ragweed pollen and/or dust mites. Although the shots can and usually do contain a mix of allergens, the more extensive the list of allergenic culprits, and the more sensitive the patient is to the various allergens, the longer it will take to obtain good protection from the shots. For example, in a simple case of ragweed allergy, generally 12 to 15 weeks of injections starting in April will protect against the next ragweed season in August. But for someone who reacts badly to half a dozen or more allergens, immunotherapy can take years.

Even after full protection is achieved, the therapy is not over. To maintain the immunity, regular booster shots are needed every three to six weeks throughout the year *indefinitely.* Otherwise, within one to three years, allergen-specific IgE antibodies will reform when you are again exposed to the allergen, and you will be back where you started.

Don't waste your time and money. Deciding to go ahead with immunotherapy requires a commitment to go the whole nine yards. Starting the shots, then stopping them in a few months, then perhaps starting up again when your symptoms get worse is wasteful and ineffective. So is being inconsistent about getting to your appointments. If during the first months of therapy too much time elapses between shots, the dose cannot be increased the next time you come in. You will, in effect, be treading water instead of making progress toward your goal of allergy control. And, once you achieve the best possible protection, if you fail to keep up with maintenance doses your allergies can come galloping back, although when this will happen is unpredictable. Remember, immunotherapy for allergy is not a cure, it's a treatment. It does not permanently erase your body's tendency to overreact to innocent proteins. But it can be highly effective at suppressing that tendency.

Are They Safe?   An estimated 10 billion allergy shots are given each year and in 99.9999 percent of cases, all that happens following a desensitizing injection is redness, itching, and perhaps a little swelling at the injection site (usually on the back of the upper arm), which disappears in a few hours or within a day or two. Antihistamines and application of ice will alleviate a bothersome local reaction. The main risk of immunotherapy is that it can sometimes trigger an allergic reaction. If the proper doses are used and administered in slowly increasing amounts, this should not happen. If there is an untoward reaction, the time between doses or the amount of allergen injected may have to be adjusted.

Very, very, very rarely, a severe and potentially life-threatening allergic reaction may occur. This is why allergists have their patients sit in the waiting room for 20 to 30 minutes after receiving desensitization shots. Should such a reaction occur, the doctor must immediately use life-saving emergency treatment to stop it. Just to give you an idea of how rare such reactions are, you are 16,000 times more likely to die in a car accident and 30 times more likely to die from being struck by lightning than from an allergy shot.

Table 11: Benefits and Risks of Allergy Treatments

No matter how safe and effective a treatment may be, it is bound to have side effects. Some side effects are experienced by most people who receive the treatment; others happen only rarely. Choosing any remedy involves a balancing act: the goal is to have the benefits clearly outweigh any expected or potential risks. In other words, you want the most relief at the lowest cost to your overall well-being. This chart will help you evaluate the relative benefits and risks of various therapies intended to prevent or treat the symptoms of nasal allergies.

Medication	Benefits	Possible Side Effects
Over-the-Counter Products		
Antihistamines	Reduce itching, runny nose and sneezing by blocking action of histamine.	Drowsiness, dizziness, dry mouth.
Topical decongestants	Shrink area blood vessels, reducing swelling. In eyes, eliminate redness.	Irritation, burning in nasal passages; sneezing. Overuse causes rebound swelling. In eyes, possible rebound redness.
Oral decongestants	Reduce swelling in nasal passages by constricting blood vessels.	Irritability, appetite suppression, insomnia.
Antihistamine/ decongestant combinations	Reduce itching, sneezing, nasal congestion by blocking histamine action and constricting blood vessels.	Drowsiness, dizziness, dry mouth, appetite suppression, irritability.

Medication	Benefits	Possible Side Effects
Prescription Drugs and Therapy		
Cromolyn sodium	Prevents allergy symptoms by inhibiting release of histamine.	Mild irritation.
Antihistamines	Relieve runny nose, sneezing, itchy nose and eyes.	Some are sedating; newer drugs are not but some may cause serious side effects if certain other drugs are also taken (see page 87).
Antihistamine/ decongestant combinations	Reduce nasal congestion, relieve sneezing and watery eyes by blocking histamine action and constricting blood vessels.	Dizziness, disturbed coordination. Sedation from antihistamine may be negated by stimulation from decongestant.
Nasal corticosteroids	Relieve itching, sneezing, and nasal blockage by inhibiting inflammatory response to allergen.	Nasal irritation and dryness, bleeding, crusting, nasal perforations.
Immunotherapy (allergy shots)	Gradually subdues reactions to inhaled allergens over period of months to years.	Time-consuming, expensive; local reactions may cause temporary discomfort; very rare risk of serious reactions.

Do Herbal Remedies Help?

Late one winter before any tree or grass had even contemplated pollinating, my brother Jeff decided to try something new to combat his annual attack of allergic rhinitis. He'd been plagued by allergies since early childhood, and he was tired of sneezing and sniffling through the spring and depending on medicines for relief. So, on the advice of a friend, he began swallowing five alfalfa tablets each morning (along with the garlic tablets to lower his cholesterol and blood pressure and vitamins for general purposes).

That spring, he says, was the least troublesome allergy season he could recall. So he kept up his remedy through the summer and, lo and behold, ragweed season was much more tolerable as well. Now Jeff is sold on alfalfa, and as long as it seems to be helping, he'll keep downing those tablets. Never mind that there are no scientific studies to support his regimen. As far as he can tell, it's working and has caused no bad side effects, and that's all that matters to him.

Herbal remedies for all sorts of health problems have become the rage among many health-conscious people. Surprisingly little herbal attention has been directed at allergic rhinitis. Even the most comprehensive books on herbal remedies mention only one or two possibilities, if any at all. There's parsley, which, according to a study published in the *Journal of Allergy and Clinical Immunology,* can inhibit the secretion of histamine. Michael Castleman, author of *100 Healing Herbs,* suggests steeping 2 teaspoons of dried parsley leaves or root (or 1 teaspoon of bruised seeds) in 1 cup of boiling water and drinking up to 3 cups of the brew each day. He warns, however, that those with sensitive skin should be wary of a possible rash caused by the psoralen in parsley.

There's honey, with its traces of pollen that a physician in Heidelberg, Germany, said helped reduce hay-fever symptoms in 84 percent of 70 allergy-prone children who drank a honey solution each day during allergy season and three times a week during the winter. Could the bits of pollen be acting as desensitizing doses, just like those in allergy shots? The physician did not do the tests needed to find out. Nor did he offer a look-alike remedy randomly assigned to a comparable group of children to see how much of the benefit he observed was simply a placebo effect—the children felt better because they believed they were taking something that would help them or as a result of the attention they received, rather than because the "treatment" had any direct benefit.

Other herbal suggestions for fighting nasal allergies have included drinking 3 to 4 cups of stinging nettle tea seasoned with 3 tablespoons of Swedish bitters; taking daily infusions or tinctures of herbs like eyebright, ground ivy, or ribwort plantain; and taking capsules of bentonite clay, wild cherry bark, mullein leaf, and horehound. The suggestions are based on hearsay, however, not science of any sort.

Perhaps the only such remedies that have at least the suggestion of a biological basis for a beneficial effect are the antioxidant nutrients, vitamins C and E and selenium. By knocking out some of the irritating oxidative pollutants like cigarette smoke and combustion fumes, these nutrients may reduce exposure to substances that can aggravate nasal allergy symptoms. Some herbal enthusiasts insist that flavonoids such as quercetin, found in many fruits and flowers, have a similar antioxidant benefit for allergy sufferers.

But the herb with the best established benefit is one used for thousands of years by the Chinese and that is the basis for a widely used drug to relieve nasal congestion. The drug is ephedrine and its original botanical source is a plant called *Ephedra sinica*. But before you choose the herbal over the pharmaceutical form of this drug, take note: it can increase blood pressure and heart rate and cause insomnia and anxiety. It should not be taken by people with heart disease, high blood pressure, thyroid disease, diabetes, or enlarged prostates. Nor should people take it who are also taking medications to lower blood pressure or combat depression. Some of the herbal formulations of ephedra contain doses that are dangerously high, perhaps even for totally healthy individuals. And the Chinese version, ma huang, has caused some severe reactions, including a number of deaths. It is the herbal remedy about which the Food and Drug Administration receives the most reports of adverse reactions, and its use may soon be banned nationwide.

If you're looking for advice on combatting your allergies, I would not recommend asking a health food store proprietor, naturopath, or self-styled herbalist. Nor would I suggest relying on the advice of friends and neighbors. Medicines, whether they come from someone's garden or the local pharmacy, all have side effects. At least with the ones from the pharmacy, you have a good chance of finding out what these effects might be *before* you take, or even buy, the remedy. Also, with drugs sold in pharmacies, you know just how much of the drug you are getting *and* how much of it you should be taking. With herbal remedies, doses are unregulated and often inaccurately stated, products may be adulterated with unknown and possibly hazardous substances (especially if the named product is costly), and even the recommended dose could be dangerously high.

When to See a Specialist

Nowadays, more and more of the functions of medical specialists are being turned over to so-called primary-care physicians—mostly family physicians, the modern-day version of the general practitioner. But however well-trained a family physician may be (they undergo postgraduate training in family medicine), there is no way he or she can know as much as a specialist would know about his or her specialty.

Knowing when to refer a patient to a specialist in allergy is as important as knowing how to treat routine cases on one's own, but the demands of managed-care plans can sometimes get in the way of an appropriate referral. Therefore, it is important for patients to know when they should be sent to a specially trained allergist and to insist on being referred when it is warranted. Allergy experts say a referral to a specialist can be helpful under the following circumstances:

- When the diagnosis is uncertain or when specialized diagnostic allergy tests—for example, skin tests—are needed.
- When a patient's symptoms are not adequately controlled and expert consultation is needed with regard to reducing environmental allergens, receiving more effective medications, or undergoing immunotherapy (allergy shots).
- When patients experience adverse effects from medication prescribed to control symptoms.
- When other related or more serious medical problems, such as asthma, chronic sinusitis, nasal polyps, fluid in the middle ear, structural abnormalities, or enlarged adenoids or tonsils, complicate the patient's condition.
- When the patient's symptoms may be due to occupational exposure, to obtain a definite diagnosis and explore ways to remedy the situation.
- When complications associated with treatment or difficulty in controlling allergy symptoms are compromising the patient's quality of life.

Appendix I

WHAT DOES IT MEAN?
AN ALLERGY GLOSSARY

Allergen: Any substance to which the body can develop an allergic reaction involving the formation of IgE antibodies. For example, pollen grains, dust mites, mold spores, and animal dander are common allergens that cause nasal allergies.

Allergenic: Capable of causing an allergic reaction.

Allergic rhinitis: Literally an allergen-caused inflammation of the nose, this allergic disorder is triggered by airborne allergens. It is characterized by both nasal and other symptoms, including sneezing; runny and/or stuffy nose; red, itchy, teary eyes; and such ancillary symptoms as fatigue, irritability, and difficulty concentrating. Allergic rhinitis can be seasonal, in response to pollen grains, or perennial, triggered by mold spores, dust mites, or animal dander.

Allergy: An immunological response to an otherwise harmless substance (allergen), resulting in the production of IgE antibodies and reactions like allergic rhinitis, asthma, hives, or swelling.

Antibody: A protein produced by the body's immunological system in response to an antigen. For example, the influenza virus, acting as an antigen, prompts the body to make anti-bodies that help to fight the infection. In allergy, the body makes antibodies to innocent substances like pollen grains and mold spores.

Anticholinergic effects: Side effects, such as excessive drying of the mouth and eyes and palpitations, that can result from treatment with antihistamines and other medications.

Antigen: A substance, usually a protein, that the body treats as foreign and that prompts it to form antibodies. In allergies, the body treats otherwise innocent substances like proteins in pollen grains and dust-mite excrement as antigens, which ultimately results in an allergic reaction. Antigens that cause allergies are called allergens.

Antihistamine: Any of a number of over-the-counter and pre-scription drugs capable of blocking or reducing the action of histamine, which is produced by immune system cells in the course of an allergic reaction and which is responsible for most of the symptoms of allergies. Some kinds of antihista-mines are sold over-the-counter (without a prescription); these tend to cause drowsiness in many users. Others are available only with a physician's prescription; these are much more expensive but most are non-sedating and equally ef-fective.

Decongestant: Any substance that can relieve nasal congestion. Medications that are decongestants tend to be stimulating and may interfere with sleep. They are sold individually or in combination with antihistamines.

Histamine: A chemical substance produced by the body and housed in the mast cells of the immune system; when released from these cells, histamine triggers the symptoms of allergies.

Hypersensitivity: An exaggerated adverse reaction to a sub-stance. For example, allergic rhinitis is caused by a hypersen-sitivity to pollens and other airborne substances that do not bother other people.

Hypoallergenic: Unlikely to cause an allergic reaction, usually referring to a product like the stuffing in pillows.

Immune response: How the body recognizes and reacts to a foreign substance, be it a bacterium, a pollen grain, or tissue from an unrelated person.

Immunoglobulin: Any of several kinds of antibodies produced by the body's immune system in response to an antigen. For example, in someone with an allergy to mold spores, the body produces immunoglobulin E, or IgE, that hooks up with the spores and starts the chain of reactions leading up to allergic symptoms.

Immunotherapy: A treatment regimen, popularly called allergy shots or desensitizing injections, that is designed to reduce the body's tendency to overreact to specific allergens.

Mast cell: A cell that is part of the body's immune system and that houses granules of histamine and other irritating chemicals. When stimulated by IgE antibody, mast cells release the contents of these granules, which trigger allergic symptoms.

Appendix II

ALLERGY INFORMATION AND PRODUCT GUIDE

TO FIND OUT MORE

The following organizations, newsletters, and information booklets and pamphlets can help you better understand allergic rhinitis and how to cope with it.

ORGANIZATIONS

- American Academy of Allergy, Asthma, and Immunology
  611 East Wells Street
  Milwaukee, WI 53202
  (414)272-6071

- National Institute of Allergy and Infectious Diseases
  31 Center Drive, MSC 2520
  Building 31, Room 7A 50
  Bethesda, MD 20892-2520
  (301)496-5717

- Asthma and Allergy Foundation of America
  1125 15th Street NW, Suite 502
  Washington, D.C. 20005
  (202)466-7643

- National Jewish Center for Immunology
  and Respiratory Medicine
  1400 Jackson Street
  Denver, CO 80206
  (303)388-4461

- American College of Allergy, Asthma, and Immunology
  85 West Algonquin Road, Suite 550
  Arlington Heights, IL 60005
  (708)427-1200
  (800)842-7777
  In addition to providing informational brochures, the college
  maintains regional listings of board-certified allergists.

NEWSLETTER

- *Asthma and Allergy Advocate*
  Published quarterly. Available free in allergists' offices or by
  subscription for $6 a year from:
  American Academy of Allergy, Asthma, and Immunology
  611 East Wells Street
  Milwaukee, WI 53202
  (414)272-6071

BOOKLETS AND PAMPHLETS, ETC.

- *Allergic Diseases*
  NIH Publication No. 91–3221
  Clinical Center Communications
  National Institutes of Health
  9000 Rockville Pike
  Building 10, Room 1C255
  Bethesda, MD 20892

- *Facts about Hay Fever*
  American Lung Association of New York
  432 Park Avenue South
  New York, NY 10016
  (Free with a self-addressed, stamped business-sized envelope.)

Note: The following materials have a commercial connection:
- *The Gardener's Guide to Allergies*
  Chlor-Trimeton Gardener's Guide
  P.O. Box 5462, Department B
  Young America, MN 55558-5462
  (Free with a self-addressed, stamped business-sized envelope.
  Offer expires September 30, 1997.)

- *Allergy Management Kit*
  Prepared by the American Lung Association and the makers
  of Tavist-1 and Tavist-D.
  Call (800)828-4783.

WHERE TO BUY IT: ALLERGY PRODUCT SOURCES

Many allergy-control products can be purchased in department stores, hardware and home products stores, and pharmacies. However, if the products you desire are not locally available, the following companies can be helpful.

- Allergy Control Products
  96 Danbury Road
  Ridgefield, CT 06877
  (800)422-DUST(3878), Monday–Friday 8:30 A.M. to 8 P.M.
  eastern time, Saturday 9:30 A.M. to 4 P.M. eastern time.

Products sold by mail order at discount prices include bedding materials, carpet-care products, face masks, vacuum cleaners and filters, mold-control products, air cleaners, and humidity-control products.

- American Allergy Supply
  P.O. Box 722022
  Houston, TX 77272
  (713)995-6110, Monday–Friday 9 A.M. to 4 P.M. central time.

Products sold by mail order include allergen-proof bed covers, air filters and cleaners, a HEPA vacuum cleaner, and Acarosan dust-mite powder.

- National Allergy Supply, Inc.
  4400 Abbotts Bridge Road
  P.O. Box 1658
  Duluth, GA 30136
  (800)522-1448

Products sold at discount prices by mail order include bedding materials, filters, a HEPA vacuum cleaner and anti-allergen dust bags, treated dust cloths, dust-mite and mold treatments, and air cleaners.

- Allergy Asthma Technology Ltd.
  P.O. Box 18398
  Chicago, IL 60618
  (800)621-5545

Products sold by mail order include bedding materials, air cleaners, dehumidifiers, air-vent filters, face masks, treated dust cloths, a HEPA vacuum cleaner, dust-mite and mold treatments, and mold-resistant shower curtains.

- Aller/Guard Inc.
  40 Cinty Lane
  Ocean, NJ 07712
  (800)234-0816

Allergy-control products sold by mail order include bedding materials and dust-mite and mildew-control products.